Fundamentals of the Stem Cell Debate

The publisher gratefully acknowledges the generous contribution to this book provided by the Barbara S. Isgur Public Affairs Endowment Fund of the University of California Press Foundation.

Fundamentals of the Stem Cell Debate

The Scientific, Religious, Ethical, and Political Issues

Edited by

Kristen Renwick Monroe,
Ronald B. Miller, and
Jerome S. Tobis

UNIVERSITY OF CALIFORNIA PRESS
Berkeley · Los Angeles · London

University of California Press, one of the most distinguished university presses in the United States, enriches
lives around the world by advancing scholarship in the
humanities, social sciences, and natural sciences. Its activities are supported by the UC Press Foundation and
by philanthropic contributions from individuals and
institutions. For more information, visit
www.ucpress.edu.

University of California Press
Berkeley and Los Angeles, California

University of California Press, Ltd.
London, England

Library of Congress Cataloging-in-Publication Data

Monroe, K. R.
    Fundamentals of the Stem Cell Debate: The Scientific,
Religious, Ethical, and Political Issues / Monroe.
        p.   cm.
    Includes bibliographical references and index.
    ISBN: 978-0-520-25210-3 (cloth : alk. paper)
    ISBN: 978-0-520-25212-7 (pbk. : alk. paper)
    1. Embryonic stem cells—Research—Moral and ethi-
cal aspects—United States.   2. Embryonic stem cells—
Research—Religious aspects—United States.
3. Embryonic stem cells—Research—Political aspects—
United States.   I. Monroe, Kristen R., 1946–
II. Miller, Ronald Baker.   III. Tobis, Jerome S., 1915–
        [DNLM: 1. Embryonic Stem Cells—United States.
2. Biomedical Research—ethics—United States.
3. Human Experimentation—ethics—United States.
4. Public Policy—United States.   QU 328 F981 2008]

QH588.S83F86   2008
174.2'8—dc22   2007031375

Manufactured in the United States of America

15   14   13   12   11   10   09   08

10   9   8   7   6   5   4   3   2   1

This book is printed on Cascades Enviro 100, a 100%
postconsumer waste, recycled, de-inked fiber. FSC recycled certified and processed chlorine free. It is acid
free, Ecologo certified, and manufactured by BioGas
energy.

To Paul H. Silverman, who pioneered work in genome and stem cell research and whose vision provided the drive behind this volume. Paul passed away July 15, 2004. We shall miss him.

Contents

Introduction: Framing the Controversy

Kristen Renwick Monroe, Ronald B. Miller, and Jerome S. Tobis

Few advances in science have generated as much excitement and public debate as the discovery of human embryonic stem cells. The potential of these cells to replace diseased or damaged cells in virtually every tissue of the body heralds the advent of an extraordinary new field of medicine that promises cures for diseases until now thought incurable. These remarkable cells, therefore, have captured the imagination of scientists and clinicians alike and have given patients a renewed sense of hope.

Controversy exists, however, because the current technique to harvest these cells involves destruction of the human blastocyst, a pre-embryo, whether obtained by in vitro fertilization or by therapeutic cloning (somatic cell nuclear transfer). Too often, debate over the use of embryonic stem cells forces discussion into two extreme positions. One camp argues that we must either allow all stem cell research all the time or consider ourselves responsible for failing to prevent the suffering and death of untold millions of human beings. The other camp argues that the use of embryonic stem cells amounts to mass murder of young life. We wish to avoid such polarizing debate, which oversimplifies complex issues, demonizes people of goodwill who hold differing opinions, and inflames rather than informs policy discussions.

We do recognize the passion in the debate, however, and our discussions in this volume respect the intensity of belief. While we do not speak for all the authors in this volume, the editors have tried to assemble chapters that recognize that the crux of the controversy depends not on an objectively derived or even a widely held scientific definition of human life but rather on a personal definition, which in many cases derives from religious faith and personal belief. Because of this, the policy debate over the use of embryonic stem cells cannot easily be resolved.

Indeed, the controversy is worldwide and many nations have entered into internal deliberation on the subject. In the United States, Congress has discussed the subject for several years; as we write, stem cell legislation has been vetoed twice by President Bush on what the president described as moral, not scientific grounds.[1] On a federal level, therefore, only rules that establish the use of federal funds for work with human embryonic stem cells have been established, and these only by presidential initiative. On a state level, the rules vary widely. For example, in California, such research is allowed but reproductive cloning is not; in some states, all human embryonic stem cell research is banned. The U.S. Congress is still considering legislation on stem cell research, and stem cells played a political role in the presidential election of 2004, as they doubtless will in the next congressional and presidential elections.

But public policies are made even in the midst of controversy, indeed, often in the midst of controversy. One could argue that the majority of issues related to science and technology—among others—are decided with a public understanding of science or facts that is far from perfect. Morality, science, and politics play no larger a role in the debate over stem cell research than they did in the public discussions over smallpox vaccination or abortion. While the hope is that improved public understanding of science will lead to better policies, this may be more useful myth than actual reality.[2] The debate over embryonic stem cells is further complicated by the lack of consensus among scientists. So the debate over the use of human embryonic stem cells is one in which both scientific and political advances move quickly, and stem cell research and its political, scientific, and ethical climate are changing rapidly. It is because of this debate that we have compiled a volume that presents a lucid discussion of the basic issues, in language that the public can understand. This volume offers a broad overview of the essential aspects of the controversy and encourages the kind of dialogue necessary to progress toward a resolution appropriate for science, medicine, patients, ethics, and public policy.

ORGANIZATION OF THE VOLUME

The stem cell controversy is framed by the late Paul H. Silverman, well-known scientist and university administrator who, with Jerome Tobis, initially proposed the conference that engendered this volume and who—unfortunately—died shortly after the conference.[3] Silverman posed the central question, for stem cells and for all scientific work with important public ramifications: Are public decisions, on an issue that touches on personal ethics and science, rooted in reason based on scientific knowledge of stem cells and on reasonable predictions? Or do individual, faith-based beliefs in the personhood or ensoulment of a fertilized cell carry the day? For Silverman, the current controversy is part of an ongoing struggle, since the time of the Enlightenment and the birth of the Age of Science, between knowledge and belief or between reason and faith. Silverman respected the individual conscience while coming down firmly in favor of reasoned discourse and scientific knowledge when matters of public policy are concerned.

In chapter 1, Peter Bryant and Philip Schwartz review the scientific knowledge of stem cells and their potential both to proliferate without differentiation and to differentiate into many, if not all, tissues. Bryant and Schwartz differentiate embryonic stem cells from adult stem cells and point out that many tissues undergo continual replacement from stem cells. They note the tremendous therapeutic potential of stem cells in replacing damaged tissues or even whole organs. Their chapter is designed to survey the current scientific knowledge of stem cells and to provide a sense of what scientists know—and what they deem controversial—in language accessible to the educated lay reader.

The next chapter, also by Schwartz and Bryant, brings a clinical perspective to the issue. The authors describe current established, therapeutic uses of stem cells for blood, immune, and metabolic disorders. They then review the experimental therapeutic use of neural stem cells for multiple sclerosis. Next, they discuss potential theoretical applications for Parkinson's disease, spinal cord injury, retinal degeneration, diabetes mellitus, brain tumors, cardiovascular disease, metabolic disorders, and osteoporosis. They discuss methods to abrogate or prevent immune rejection, which greatly complicates stem cell therapy if the cells are not genetically identical to the recipient. They conclude with discussion of scientific and ethical issues arising in stem cell therapy. These two chapters lay the foundation for understanding the scientific issues and the clinical possibilities of stem cell research.

Much of the controversy over stem cell research emanates from religious or ethical beliefs concerning the origin of life. Rather than adopt either an adversarial position or one of advocacy, we chose to follow Silverman's admonition to address issues of science and religion in a careful, scholarly way. In chapter 3, Mahtab Jafari, Fanny Elahi, Saba Ozyurt, and Ted Wrigley thus survey the major world religions and ask what each religion suggests about the origin of life and how this position relates to broader issues concerning scientific research, including research on stem cells. Jointly written by medical scientists and social scientists, this chapter addresses what may be the most controversial questions concerning stem cell research: When does life begin, and how do our views on that question influence our decisions about stem cell research? The authors examine the views of the major religions concerning the origin of life and suggest how one's position on these important, and highly charged, questions affects a wide range of issues concerning scientific work. The chapter is important for two reasons. First, it offers a dispassionate analysis of the various religious views, and second, it broadens the discussion, moving away from the contrast between fundamentalist Christian religion and a "scientific" view to include a comparative, worldwide religious perspective.

Philip Nickel presents the view of a philosopher and ethicist concerned with the ethical issues surrounding stem cell research. In particular, Nickel focuses on what he views as largely symbolic, but nonetheless highly charged, issues: the loss of potential future human life and the moral standing or dignity of the embryo. Nickel argues that the critical issues are not moral but rather are couched in statistical and political terms: How many people support stem cell research, and how many oppose or are disgusted by embryonic stem cell research? Nickel's chapter provides a nice segue to what seems to be shaping up as the crux of the debate over stem cell research: politics.

The next two chapters of the volume are devoted to the politics of stem cell research. Larry Goldstein discusses stem cell politics prior to the passage of Proposition 71, the California Stem Cell Research and Cures Act. His is the view of a scientist in the trenches and a public-minded citizen-advisor of legislators. Goldstein takes the position that his responsibility as a physician-scientist to present and future patients with disorders potentially treatable with stem cells outweighs his responsibility to the early human embryo. He also points out that stem cell research with human embryonic stem cells may allow an understanding of human disease not currently possible from animal research. Finally, Goldstein discusses the greater value of public funding of scientific research as compared with private funding, since public funding ensures public scrutiny of research. Further, he suggests that we cannot avoid the difficult moral choice by studying only adult stem cells because they may not have the same potential as embryonic stem cells. He concludes that the policy issues (moral, legal, and social) of stem cell research must be decided—as they are for other controversial issues that affect society—by the democratic process.

Lee Zwanziger, a scientist-historian-philosopher, considers the politics of stem cell research from a national perspective. Zwanziger also discusses the importance of public funding for the oversight of research. However, she believes agreement probably cannot be achieved simply by greater public education about the scientific aspects of stem cell research and technology because not all disagreement is due to ignorance of the science. Rather, there is basic disagreement about the nature and moral status of the early embryo, and this precludes agreement at least in the near future simply by further public discourse or by democratic policy decision making. Further, Zwanziger is not convinced that we need a uniform national policy given the substantially different views that have already been expressed by different states.

The chapters by Goldstein and Zwanziger describe the intensity of the debate as it existed at the time of the initial conference, in May 2004, at which several of these papers were presented.[4] These chapters locate the controversy in politics, not science. In the last chapters, Sidney Golub and Ronald Miller offer a synthetic analysis of the debate. Golub's chapter provides a current summary of federal, international, and state politics relative to human embryonic stem cells. It begins by reviewing federal legislation and regulation and the current impasse both in providing federal support of human embryonic stem cell research and in passing legislation that would ban cloning. Golub then reviews failed international treaty efforts and the inability to agree even on a ban of reproductive cloning. Finally, Golub reviews the variably enabling and restricting legislation and regulation by different states. He predicts less federal and more state funding and regulation of human embryonic stem cell research in the future.

The final chapter, by Ronald B. Miller, serves as a summary of the ethical issues in stem cell research, therapy, and public policy. Miller begins with a brief recapitulation of normal embryologic development and the sources of stem cells and then quotes a statement of ethical goals for stem cell research. Next he reviews two issues of general societal agreement and two of major societal disagreement that complicate, if not prevent, the development of satisfactory public policy. He then recapitulates the religious as well as secular ethical beliefs and concepts fundamental to a concluding overview of the ethical issues for stem cell research, stem cell therapy, and stem cell policy development. He reviews the several scientific strategies for obtaining potent human stem cells that have been proposed to avoid critical ethical objections. In conclusion, Miller quotes opinions regarding whether we can achieve societal consensus and possible approaches for doing so.

PURPOSE OF THE VOLUME

The debate over stem cell research is complex and complicated by divergent religious views and by electoral politics. Our purpose in this volume is to present the major issues dispassionately, as a careful scientist presents them, raising the complexities and controversies but doing so in a manner that is accessible to the general public, since ultimately stem cell research will be critically influenced, if not decided, by public policies.

The issues raised here thus are important and of concern not just to scientists and potential patients but also to the public. Does stem cell research destroy human life? If so, is embryonic stem cell research justified for broader humanitarian reasons? How will public decisions be made, and what role will faith and science play in the decision making? Is there sufficient scientific evidence of clinical benefit (or lack thereof) to justify political or policy decisions that promote or limit stem cell research? Do we not need more basic and applied research before such decisions are made? How will scientific research respond to the extant political realities and restrictions on embryonic stem cell research?

While these are perhaps the major questions of the debate, other questions also arise, and we hope readers will think of some of these issues as they read the chapters that follow. Who owns the intellectual property associated with stem cell research? How should the public receive a return on its investment in stem cell research? Should genes be patented? What will happen to the frozen embryos left over from in vitro fertilization if they are not used for embryonic stem cell research? Are the Roman and the American Catholic Church in agreement on these matters? Does the Hippocratic tradition of doing no harm preclude embryonic stem cell research? What is the moral status of a parthenogenetic blastocyst, a blastocyst or early embryo derived from an unfertilized egg stimulated artificially to develop into an organism rather than one derived from a sperm-fertilized egg? The parthogenote then is an organism derived from a single individual rather than from two individuals or "parents." Can we reframe the public and scientific discussion to avoid language that polarizes the debate unnecessarily? Is the word *embryo* itself unnecessarily polarizing? Is it scientifically precise? Is it useful to speak of a *pre-embryo*? What about the term *therapeutic cloning*? Should we speak of *somatic cell nuclear transfer* rather than *cloning* when we wish to generate new stem cell lines? Or is this language simply too technical and unwieldy for public discourse?

The contributors to this volume differ on several critical points, but all agree that the first step toward good public policy is scientific knowledge. As Zwanziger notes in chapter 6 of this book, failing to understand the science will result in bad debate and can lead to bad policy, but understanding the science is not sufficient to ensure wisdom in either. The difficulty is whether disagreement comes from ignorance of the facts or from different interpretation of the meaning of the facts. We hope this volume will contribute to increased public awareness of the scientific facts and that such awareness will lead to more informed public opinion and public policies concerning this important issue.

NOTES

1. The developments in this area move so quickly that some of what we now write will surely be out of date. See the op-ed by Deborah Blum, "A Pox on Stem Cell Research," *New York Times,* A19, August 1, 2006, or Nicholas Wade's "Some Scientists See Shift in Stem Cell Hopes," *New York Times,* August 14, 2006, A18.

2. See work on science technology by B. Wynne among others, or Blum, "Pox on Stem Cell Research," for a discussion of the debate over smallpox.

3. Paul's was a passionate life in science, from his first research into malaria vaccine to his work on the Human Genome Project. Paul established the nation's first human genome center in 1987 at the Lawrence Berkeley National Laboratory and later worked in university administrations to further scientific discoveries. He served as the provost for research and graduate studies at the State University of New York and as president of the University of Maine. He then moved to the University of California at Berkeley, where he held a number of positions, eventually becoming director of the Biotechnology Research and Education Program for all the University of California campuses. His last official position was as associate vice chancellor for the health sciences at UC Irvine.

We remember Paul as a Renaissance man who lived at the cutting edge of scientific issues, even when these issues were controversial. This volume reflects Paul's conviction that the public can make wise choices if advances in science and technology are explained in clear and understandable language. We have tried to honor Paul by following his lead in this volume, explaining the scientific issues in language designed to be accessible to the educated lay reader. While the volume attempts to present a balanced perspective, including a variety of scholarly opinions, we also wish to honor Paul's passion about stem cell research by noting his strong advocacy for broadening the use of this technique. Paul's last public remarks on this topic convey some of the fervor of his convictions on this subject.

Paul argued, shortly before his death, that the "discovery of accessible human stem cells and the subsequent research focused on clinical application inadvertently provoked an intersection of conflicting religious, philosophical, political, scientific, and secular systems of belief." In editing Paul's remarks, the editors have tried to retain the passion of Paul's original piece while integrating it into a volume that underwent significant editorial revision in response to the kind of scholarly debate Paul so cherished. The editors appreciate the comments of the other contributors, the anonymous reviewers, Ted Wrigley's assistance in modifying this document, and Nancy Silverman's permission to publish it.

Paul linked many of the issues that arose as part of this debate to arguments characteristic of the intense emotional debates of the seventeenth and eighteenth centuries, when the Roman Catholic and Reformation churches reacted negatively to the rational explanations of natural phenomena provided by scientific processes. Paul felt that stem cell research and its potential application to the treatment of a variety of incurable human illness have been greatly hampered by political and judicial actions in several countries.

The United States, Germany, and France are but several prominent examples of this phenomenon. For example, in the United States, President Bush announced on August 9th, 2001, that scientists in the United States receiving federal funding were proscribed from using new cell lines that might be obtained from frozen fertilized eggs that were initially the by-product of in vitro fertilization procedures and were scheduled to be discarded. This left only the sixty or so stem cell lines already established. About four hundred thousand of these embryos were estimated to be available in 2001, though many of those available were spoken for, and only a small proportion could have been turned into viable stem cell lines. The announcement was accompanied by language concerning sacredness of human life and the significant moral hazards implicit in stem cell research and was promoted by the group of Evangelical Christian congressional delegates.

In my view, this policy places severe limits on university scientists and laboratories supported by funding from the National Institutes of Health. This constitutes a significant portion of the research in the field. The proscription remains in place even in spite of appeals from other conservatives, such as Strom Thurmond, Orrin Hatch, and, very recently, Nancy Reagan.

As a result of the president's religious beliefs, then, science administrative positions, advisory groups, and the judiciary are being filled with people who have been active in advancing the religious understanding that the soul enters the egg at the time of fertilization. This belief system has accounted for the numerous legislative and judicial attempts to confer "personhood" even on the earliest multicell embryos—the blastocysts, which contain the 120 harvestable stem cells [see chapter 1 of this book]—to grant them legal protection against scientific experimentation. Some proposed legislation carries severe criminal penalties.

However, as is often the case, events have overtaken the concepts and thinking of those who would declare criminals of those who might establish stem cell lines for study and experimentation. The cloning of Dolly the sheep by somatic cell nuclear transfer (not fertilization) in 1997 demonstrated that the DNA nuclear hereditary material from a highly specialized mammary gland cell can be reprogrammed to become a totipotent embryonic stem cell capable of producing all of the more than two hundred cell types required to make up a sheep's body. The cloning of Dolly suggested that any cell in the body can be reprogrammed to become another individual. Cloning by somatic cell nuclear transfer has now been accomplished repeatedly and efficiently in cattle, pigs, mice, and rats. Researchers at the University of Pennsylvania have accomplished a remarkable transformation in in vitro cultures by converting a specialized cell into a stem cell and then stimulating it to become a producer of sperm. This has now been accomplished in vivo by the dedifferentiation of specialized cells into germline stem cells (*Science*, May 14, 2006). The significance of these developments is that—theoretically, and soon practically—any of the ten trillion cells in the human body, under appropriate conditions, can be converted into a potential human. The newly discovered plasticity of the human genome is opening up new opportunities for regeneration and repair of diseased tissue.

Paul believed scientific reasoning and objectivity could alter strongly held belief systems. One of his desires in proposing and crafting this volume was to remind people that we live in a pluralistic, multicultural society, with tolerance and respect for different worldviews. His hope was that the debate in this volume would encourage public policies and public policy debate based on such principles.

4. The conference was sponsored by the University of California, Irvine (UCI) Interdisciplinary Center for the Scientific Study of Ethics and Morality, in co-sponsorship with the UCI's Newkirk Center for Science and Society, Institute for Genomics and Bioinformatics, Schools of Biological Science, Social Science, Social Ecology, Medicine, Humanities, and Information and Computer Science, Henry Samueli School of Engineering, and Paul Merage School of Management; the Children's Hospital of Orange County; and the UCI Dialogue Society. We appreciate their support and that of Bettye Vaughen and Frank Lynch, who contributed to the production of this volume. None of the individuals or institutions acknowledged here, however, is responsible for the views expressed in this volume.

CHAPTER I

Stem Cells

Peter J. Bryant and Philip H. Schwartz

WHAT ARE STEM CELLS?

Stem cells are undifferentiated cells found in the embryos and the later life stages of animals, including humans. They are recognized by their dualistic nature: they either can expand their numbers (self-renew) while remaining undifferentiated or can differentiate and contribute to the development or repair of tissues of the body. Some authors have added other criteria to the definition, including the ability to produce cells differentiating in different ways (multipotency); the ability of a single cell to proliferate into a population of similar cells (clone-forming ability); and the ability to keep dividing indefinitely (unlimited proliferative capacity)—the latter property distinguishing them from most other noncancerous cell types, which can undergo only a limited number of divisions. In most examples of stem cells only some of these properties have been demonstrated, and the term *stem cell* has been used fairly loosely. However, stem cells of many types are now being intensively studied by genetic and molecular methods, and biologists are developing more rigorous and convenient methods to identify them. They are recognized by their expression of certain genes, their production of characteristic proteins and antigens, and their responsiveness to certain growth factors.

In the best-analyzed examples of stem cells in experimental organisms, self-renewal is accomplished through conventional symmetric cell division (figure 1), whereas differentiation is controlled through a specialized

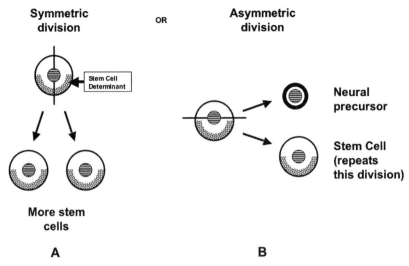

Figure 1. The fundamental characteristics of stem cells: *(A)*, Symmetric cell division leads to self-renewal of stem cells; *(B)*, Asymmetric cell division leads to replacement of the stem cell and production of a sister cell, exemplified here by a neural precursor, which may differentiate immediately or after one or a few divisions. Specifically expressed and localized stem cell determinants dictate the fate of the daughter cells.

mechanism called asymmetric cell division (ACD; figure 1). ACD results in the budding of a (usually) smaller cell from the larger stem cell (Potten 1997). Through this division the stem cell renews itself and can undergo more such divisions, while the other cell either begins to differentiate or undergoes a small number of additional divisions before the resulting cells differentiate.

When a cell begins the process of ACD, one set of specialized proteins accumulates on one side of the cell and another set accumulates on the other (figure 2). These proteins (and some messenger RNAs) are then included either in the stem cell or in the differentiating cell. Furthermore, experimental studies show that these localized molecules actually control whether the cell receiving them remains a stem cell or begins differentiating. The molecules are therefore called ACD determinants. Most of them have been identified through genetic studies of ACD during the development of the nervous system in the fruit fly *Drosophila*. In the absence of any one of the ACD determinants the asymmetry of division is disrupted, and this leads to abnormal cell proliferation and/or abnormal cell fates. Some of the ACD determinants control the localization of

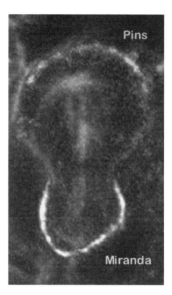

Figure 2. Fluorescently labeled ACD determinants during division of a neural stem cell in a fly embryo, showing the opposite localizations for ACD determinants in the stem cell and differentiating cell. The Miranda protein, stained red, marks the basal complex that determines the differentiating neural precursor and also includes Staufen, Prospero, Prospero mRNA, Numb, and Pon. The Pins protein, stained green, identifies the apical complex that determines the neural stem cell and also includes Atypical PKC, Gαi, Bazooka, and Insc. Image from Chris Doe, University of Oregon.

others, and the molecular interactions between them are under active study (Matsuzaki 2000).

Most of the proteins implicated in ACD in *Drosophila* have remarkably close mammalian and human counterparts (homologs), but there is only fragmentary evidence regarding the possible roles of these homologs in the control and division of mammalian stem cells. Much of the information comes from work on the formation of the nervous system in the mammalian embryo, where ACD has been demonstrated in the mouse (Shen et al. 2002) and ferret (Chenn and McConnell 1995). Preliminary studies have suggested that ACD during mammalian development is controlled by the homologs of some of the ACD determinants identified in *Drosophila*, including those named Numb, Numblike, Notch1 (Fang and Xu 2001; Justice and Jan 2002; Zhong et al. 1997; Zhong et al. 1996), and LGN (homolog of *Drosophila* Pins; Fuja et al. 2004; Mochizuki et al. 1996). In one of the most definitive studies, stem cells were isolated from the living embryonic mouse brain and cultured through a division cycle, and the resulting cell pairs were stained using antibodies against the Numb protein (Shen et al. 2002). The protein often accumulated in one of the two daughter cells, and this accumulation was correlated with the subsequent fates of the daughter cells. The Notch signaling pathway, identified genetically in *Drosophila,* also seems to be involved in ACD of satellite cells during mammalian muscle development (Conboy and Rando 2002).

The fate of stem cells as well as the way they divide appears to be a function of their microenvironment, which in many cases is provided by a specialized structure known as the stem cell niche. At least in the hematopoietic (blood cell–forming) system, the niche develops independently and the stem cells migrate to and colonize the niche (Schofield 1983). It has been suggested that the niche controls the phenotype of the stem cell, including whether it undergoes self-renewal or ACD. Evidence suggesting the existence of stem cell niches has also been obtained for the epidermis, intestinal epithelium, nervous system, and gonads (Fuchs, Tumbar, and Guasch 2004), as well as in developing muscles (Venters and Ordahl 2005). Furthermore, some of the soluble growth factors mediating interaction between niche and stem cells have been identified (Hauwel, Furon, and Gasque 2005).

EMBRYONIC STEM CELLS (ESCS)

In the mammalian embryo, following fertilization of the egg by a sperm, several cell divisions take place without any growth in total volume (figure 3), so the cells (now called blastomeres) get progressively smaller. They also rearrange to form a hollow sphere of cells (blastocyst) surrounding a fluid-filled cavity called the blastocoel. The cells of the blastocyst then segregate into an outer layer, called the trophectoderm, and an inner cell mass (ICM). The cells of the trophectoderm (trophoblasts) become the fetal contribution to the placenta, while the ICM contains the embryonic stem cells (ESCs) that give rise to the tissues of the fetus (figure 4).

Isolation

Human ESCs (hESCs) are usually obtained from the ICM of embryos produced by in vitro fertilization (IVF). In this procedure, eggs are harvested

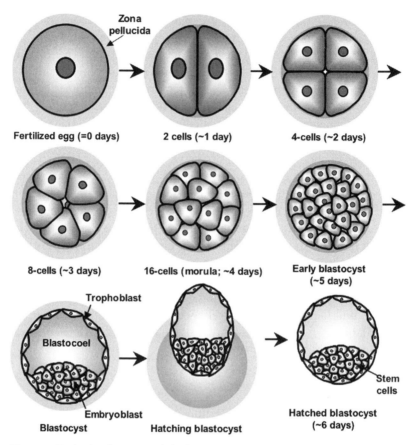

Figure 3. Early development of the human embryo. Embryonic stem cells are derived from the inner cell mass of the blastocyst. See text for explanation.

from a woman after she has been treated with follicular hormones to stimulate the ovaries. The eggs are fertilized either by combining them with sperm in a dish or by mechanically injecting the sperm into the egg (intracytoplasmic sperm injection). The latter technique has the advantage that every egg gets fertilized and that only one sperm enters each egg. The fertilized eggs are then incubated to allow them to develop into blastocysts. Then the trophectoderm is removed and the ICM is plated on to a "feeder layer" of mouse or human embryonic fibroblasts (Thomson et al. 1998), which is essential for the survival of the ICM (Cowan et al. 2004). The ICM then flattens into a compact colony of ESCs. ESC colonies are then

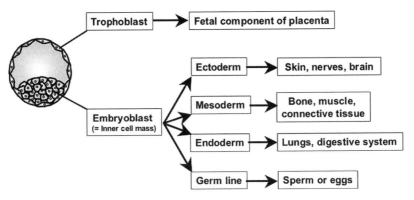

Figure 4. Products of the different cell types of the early blastocyst. The cells of the trophoblast give rise to the fetal component of the placenta, while the inner cell mass, the embryoblast, gives rise to every cell type and organ system of the body.

mechanically dissociated and replated several times to give rise to stable cell lines.

Properties

Under certain conditions hESCs can divide indefinitely while undifferentiated, but under other conditions they can differentiate into virtually any cell type in the body (Amit et al. 2000; Bodnar et al. 2004; Cowan et al. 2004; Odorico, Kaufman, and Thomson 2001; Thomson et al. 1998). When undifferentiated hESCs are transplanted into an animal, they often form a type of tumor called a teratoma (Altaba, Sanchez, and Dahmane 2002), which is unusual in that it contains cells representing all three germ layers (Trounson 2004). Indeed, the ability of hESCs to form a teratoma after injection is the accepted criterion for identifying hESCs as such.

When cultured in the laboratory, hESCs grow as compact colonies and usually require the presence of "feeder cells" for their survival (figure 5). The feeder cells are typically mouse fibroblasts that have been treated with mitotic inhibitors to prevent their proliferation. But to make hESCs safe for use in human cell therapy, methods are being developed in which the human cells have no contact with animal cells. Human feeder cells can be effective (Amit et al. 2000). Another possibility is to first condition the culture medium by incubating it with feeder cells, then

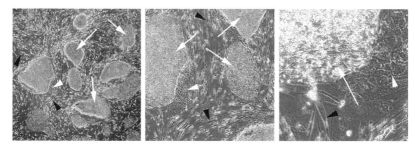

Figure 5. Human embryonic stem cells in culture. Phase-contrast photomicrographs taken at *(A)* 40x, *(B)* 100x, and *(C)* 400x magnification. Human ESCs appear as colonies of cells (white arrows) that are so tightly packed that individual cells are very difficult to discern, even at high magnification. The colonies are grown in the presence of a feeder layer of cells, in this case mouse embryonic fibroblasts (black arrowheads). Even when hESCs are grown under conditions that do not favor differentiation, they spontaneously differentiate and are then seen as groups of less tightly packed cells emanating from the sides of the colonies (white arrowheads).

remove the feeder cells and use the conditioned medium, presumably containing appropriate growth factors, for culturing the stem cells (Carpenter et al. 2004; Rosler et al. 2004; Xu et al. 2001).

Human ESCs have specific requirements for nutrients, including "serum replacement medium." Serum is a necessary component for survival and/or differentiation of many cell types, but it invariably induces differentiation of hESCs, so it cannot be used to promote their survival and/or proliferation. This problem has been overcome by the use of serum replacement medium, which has many of the supportive properties of serum but lacks the tendency to cause differentiation. Another feature of hESCs is their inability to divide and/or survive in low-density culture. When they are dissociated into a single cell suspension, these cells have a very low survival rate. Colonies are therefore usually mechanically dissected into smaller colonies, rather than dissociated into single cells, for propagation.

Human ESCs in culture have a specific morphology, and they express characteristic surface antigens and nuclear transcription factors. The surface antigens include the stage-specific embryonic antigen SSEA-4 and the teratocarcinoma recognition antigens TRA-1–60 and TRA-1–81 (Carpenter et al. 2004). The transcription factors include the POU (pit-oct-unc)-domain transcription factor Octamer-4 (Oct-4), associated with the expression of particular elements of the embryonic genome (Thomson et al. 1998).

Differentiation

When undifferentiated hESC colonies are detached from the feeder layer and transferred into serum-containing medium, they form multicellular aggregates called embryoid bodies (EBs, figure 6), which can contain cell types representing all three germ layers of the body—endoderm, mesoderm, and ectoderm (figure 4). Many EBs tend to show cell types of only one or two germ layers, but in an unpredictable manner. Thus, with appropriate subculture conditions and physical removal of colonies showing specific morphologies, behaviors, or proteins, it is possible to establish cultures that are enriched for particular cell types or mixtures of cell types (figure 6; Carpenter et al. 2004). However, this cell behavior is unpredictable and the sorting is not completely effective. Many labs have therefore been trying to develop protocols for directly controlling the differentiation of hESCs.

Exogenous differentiating factors have been useful in favoring differentiation into specific derivatives: retinoic acid and nerve growth factor for neuronal differentiation (Schuldiner et al. 2001); basic fibroblast growth factor and platelet-derived growth factor for glial precursors (Brustle et al. 1999); 5-aza-2'-deoxycytidine for cardiomyocytes (Xu et al. 2002); bone

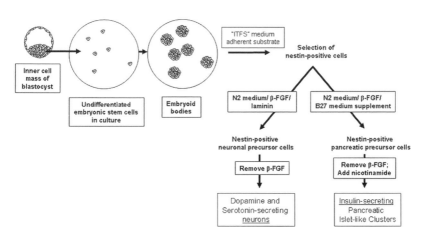

Figure 6. Harvesting and in vitro culture of embryonic stem cells for therapeutic use. Colonies of hESCs may be first differentiated into embryoid bodies, then encouraged to differentiate with specific media, selected according to the expression of specific proteins, behavior, or morphology, and then cultured using specific protocols to give rise to selected populations useful for a particular therapeutic application (Carpenter et al. 2004; He et al. 2003; Nistor et al. 2005; Perrier et al. 2004).

morphogenetic protein-4 and transforming growth factor-beta for trophoblast cells (Carpenter, Rosler, and Rao 2003); sodium butyrate for hepatocytes (Rambhatla et al. 2003); and various cytokines for hematopoietic cells (Zhan et al. 2004). Differentiation into particular tissue types can
also be elicited by overexpressing genes encoding transcription factors that
function in cell commitment during normal development: MyoD1 for
skeletal muscle (Dekel et al. 1992) and Nurr1 for dopamine neurons (Kim
et al. 2002). However, these methods still usually give only enrichment
rather than total induction, so additional sorting is often necessary. This
has been done on the basis of lineage-specific gene expression: PS-NCAM
and A2B5 as cell-surface markers for neural precursors (Carpenter et al.
2001), or hygromycin resistance driven by a myosin heavy chain promoter
for cardiomyocytes (Klug et al. 1996) (figure 6).

Several groups (Brustle et al. 1999; Reubinoff et al. 2001; Tabar et al.
2005; Wernig et al. 2004) have produced neuronal precursors from either mouse or human ESCs and tested them by injection into the developing brain of newborn mouse or embryonic rat. The transplanted cells
were incorporated into the host brain, migrated along appropriate
tracks, differentiated into neurons in a region-specific manner, and made
synaptic contacts with host neurons. In some cases the transplanted cells
also gave rise to glia and astrocytes. This procedure has been shown to
promote recovery in animal models of Parkinson's disease and spinal
cord injury (Shufaro and Reubinoff 2004).

NEURAL CREST STEM CELLS

A peculiar and heterogeneous population of migratory precursor cells,
called neural crest cells, originates during fetal development from the neural folds at the dorsal side of the neural tube. These cells migrate through
the embryo to differentiate into a bewildering collection of derivatives, including most of the neurons, Schwann cells, and glia of the peripheral nervous system; most primary sensory neurons; some endocrine cells in the
adrenal and thyroid glands; smooth muscle associated with the heart and
great vessels; pigment cells of the skin and internal organs; and bone, cartilage, and connective tissue of the face and neck (Le Douarin and Dupin
2003). The migrating cells include multipotential neural crest stem cells,
but the population becomes progressively restricted, and terminal differentiation usually ensues soon after the cells reach their targets (Baroffio,
Dupin, and Le Douarin 1991). However, some studies show that neural
crest–derived stem cells can still be identified in adult organs, including the

central nervous system (Altman 1969; Doetsch et al. 1999; Eriksson et al. 1998; Gould et al. 1999; Johansson et al. 1999; Palmer, Takahashi, and Gage 1997; Reynolds, Tetzlaff, and Weiss 1992) and the hair follicle (Sieber-Blum et al. 2004). Some of the other reported examples of adult stem cells, described below, have not yet been adequately tested to see whether they might also have a neural crest origin. Neural crest–derived cells can be identified by the expression of the neural crest marker Sox-10 (Sieber-Blum et al. 2004).

ADULT STEM CELLS

Classical embryologists developed the concept that, as mammals developed, their cells became progressively more determined for a certain tissue fate and the tissues progressively lost the potential for repair or regeneration. However, recent work has shown that many mammalian tissues contain stem cells that can mobilize, proliferate, and differentiate in response to wounding or disease. These cells can be isolated and grown in culture, and during propagation they retain the ability to differentiate into one or a few tissue types appropriate to their original site. Their potential for self-renewal, their multipotentiality, and their lack of differentiation until they receive the appropriate environmental signals have led to their designation as adult stem cells, although they are sometimes designated more conservatively as progenitor cells. They are referred to as adult stem cells to distinguish them from embryonic stem cells, even if they are taken from fetal or neonatal sources.

Adult stem cells appear to be involved in the normal tissue renewal that occurs in many organ systems, including bone marrow, skin, gut lining, blood vessels, heart, kidney, endocrine glands, liver, pancreas, mammary gland, prostate, lung, retina, and parts of the nervous system (Sell 2003). Some of the stem cell populations also appear to be able to "transdifferentiate" into other tissue types depending on their location in the body. These findings, of course, raise tremendous possibilities for cell-based therapy of many disorders, especially those involving tissue losses.

Bone Marrow: Hematopoietic Stem Cells

Bone marrow contains some of the most complex, but nevertheless best-understood, stem cell populations in the body, including the cell populations responsible for maintaining blood cells, which constitute one of the most rapidly replaced tissues in the body. Most circulating blood

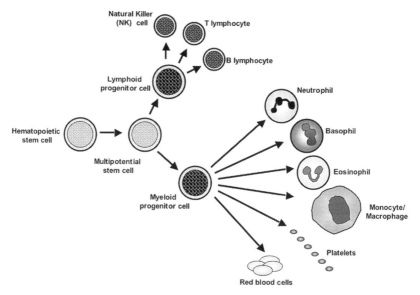

Figure 7. Bone marrow is the source of hematopoietic stem cells. This well-understood stem cell type gives rise to red blood cells and platelets as well as white blood cells (B cells and T cells) that function in the immune system.

cells cannot proliferate, so replacement of blood cells is dependent on the activity of precursors in the bone marrow (and elsewhere) called hematopoietic stem cells (Ponting, Zhao, and Anderson 2003). In a process called hematopoiesis, the stem cells give rise to several blood cell populations, including erythrocytes (red blood cells), leukocytes (white blood cells, including neutrophils, eosinophils, and basophils), monocytes, and platelets (figure 7). The bone marrow also produces all of the cells of the immune system, including B cells for the circulation and the lymph nodes and spleen; T cells for the thymus; and macrophages and dendritic cells.

The complex cell production machinery in the bone marrow involves several stem cell populations with intermediate levels of multipotency, and many of the lineage relationships between these different levels of progenitors have been worked out, but some remain hypothetical (Sell 2003). At an early point in the pathway, progenitor cells have been shown to undergo ACD in which one of the two daughters retains stem-cell properties and the other shows restriction to a smaller range of differentiation potential (Takano et al. 2004).

Bone Marrow: Mesenchymal Stem Cells

In addition to the hematopoietic system, bone marrow contains a supporting tissue called stroma. This was originally thought to simply provide a structural framework for the hematopoietic system, but it has now been found to contain several cell types with other functions and potentials. Most importantly, it contains a population of mesenchymal stem cells (MSCs; Dennis and Caplan 2003), which are strongly adherent and can therefore be isolated by culturing marrow on an appropriate substrate and washing other cells off. MSCs can give rise to many kinds of connective tissue cells, including those responsible for remodeling of cartilage, bone, fat, and vascular tissue (Pittenger et al. 1999). They also produce the essential microenvironment necessary to support the hematopoietic stem cells in the bone marrow (Dennis and Caplan 2003).

The results of bone marrow transplantation studies have led to the conclusion that this remarkable tissue can also produce cells that can circulate to various other sites in the body and contribute to even more tissues, including endothelium, muscle, liver, pancreatic islets, heart, brain, lung, kidney, and retina (Huttmann, Li, and Duhrsen 2003; Sell 2003). Some of this evidence comes from postmortem studies on women who had received bone marrow transplants from male donors. The presence of a Y chromosome provided a reliable marker for cells from the donor, even when the cells were present only in very small numbers. These studies showed evidence for bone marrow cells producing neurons in the brain (Mezey et al. 2003), as well as cells in the liver and buccal epithelium (Theise et al. 2000). Similar studies, using markers recognizing either the X or the Y chromosome, showed that bone marrow could contribute to muscle cells in the heart (Thiele et al. 2002). However, whether these cells functioned appropriately for the new site could not be determined from these studies.

Experimental studies on mice have also suggested that cells from transplanted bone marrow can contribute to other tissues, including the epithelia of the gastrointestinal and respiratory systems (Krause and Gehring 1989), skeletal muscle (Gussoni et al. 1999), heart muscle, endothelium and smooth muscle (Orlic et al. 2001), and liver (Lagasse et al. 2000; Petersen et al. 1999; Wang et al. 2003). In the studies on contribution of transplanted bone marrow to infarcted heart muscle, it has been shown by several laboratories that the damaged tissue is repaired and that heart function is improved (Mathur and Martin 2004). In most of the other cases, as with the human studies, it is not clear whether the transformed bone marrow cells improve the function of the organ in which they reside.

Some of the results in mice may reflect the directed change in the differentiation program of the bone marrow–derived cells by the tissue microenvironment. However, at least in the case of liver and muscle, some of the differentiated products from bone marrow cell transplantation may be derived by fusion of the transplanted cells with differentiated tissue cells of the host, rather than by directed differentiation of the transplanted cells. It is also possible in some cases that the transplanted bone marrow may not have been a pure cell population but may have included some stem cells of different potential. For example, it may have included multipotential MSCs or some tissue-specific stem cells that had circulated from mature organs into the bone marrow. Finally, in the studies showing improved heart function following bone marrow transplantation, much of the improvement may have been due to stimulation of the formation of new blood vessels rather than the direct contribution of the transplanted cells to muscle regeneration (Mathur and Martin 2004).

In the transplantation studies it is usually difficult to identify the factors controlling the differentiation of the transplanted cells. However, it has recently been shown that appropriate combinations of growth factors can cause the efficient conversion of stromal cells from human adult bone marrow into a population closely resembling neural stem cells (Hermann et al. 2004), which are described below. The transformed cells grow as balls called neurospheres, express neural-specific genes at high levels, and differentiate into the three main derivatives of neural stem cells: neurons (nerve cells), astrocytes (star-shaped cells with a variety of functions), and oligodendrocytes (which are responsible for generating the myelin sheath that surrounds the axons of neurons). The discovery of this expanded potential of bone marrow cells could open up many important new avenues for stem cell therapy, using a patient's own bone marrow as a convenient source of genetically compatible cells.

Liver Hematopoietic Stem Cells

The liver is the major site of blood cell formation in the mammalian embryo. Stem cells isolated from this site proved to be capable of remarkable transdifferentiation into myocytes (muscle precursor cells) following transplantation into a mouse heart that had been subjected to a myocardial infarction (Lanza et al. 2004). In this experiment the stem cells had been modified by nuclear transfer so that they were genetically identical to the host and were therefore not recognized as foreign by the host immune system. The transplanted cells contributed substantially to regeneration of the heart muscle, and the regenerated muscle replaced 38 percent of the scar after one month. Furthermore, in this report, unlike many of the reports with bone marrow transplantation, the transplanted cells appear to have clearly transformed into heart muscle, and this did not involve fusion with host muscle cells. The transplanted cells also contributed directly to the formation of new blood vessels, which connected to the host circulatory system and functioned normally. The beneficial effects on heart muscle regeneration obtained in this study were far superior to those obtained with bone marrow transplantation, suggesting that further studies on the properties of fetal liver stem cells would be very worthwhile.

Neural Stem Cells

Neural stem cells, defined by their clone-forming ability, self-renewal capability, and multipotency, were first isolated from embryonic and adult mice (Reynolds and Weiss 1996), and their origin during development (Temple 2001) and distribution in the adult (Garcia-Verdugo et al. 1998; Morshead et al. 1994) has since been analyzed in detail. Similar cells have been found in fetal, neonatal, and adult human brains (Palmer et al. 2001), where they are localized in the hippocampus and subventricular zone (SVZ) in stem cell niches (Doetsch 2003). Up to 100 million cells can easily be harvested from a single human neonatal brain (P. Schwartz et al. 2003), and these can easily be proliferated thirty-thousand-fold, yielding 3×10^{12} cells from a single brain. Single neural progenitor cells divide and, in the absence of a substrate, gradually grow into balls of 10,000 to 15,000 undifferentiated cells called neurospheres. Neural precursor cells migrate out from the neurospheres (figure 8) and can give rise to neurons, astrocytes, and oligodendrocytes (Brewer and Cotman 1989; Gage 1998; McKay 1997; Palmer et al. 2001; P. Schwartz et al. 2003; Uchida et al. 2000; Zhang et al. 2001).

The presence of neural stem cells in the adult brain accounts for the finding that neurons are generated constantly, even into adulthood, in many regions of the brain, including the SVZ of the anterior lateral ventricles and the dentate gyrus of the hippocampus (Chiasson et al. 1999; Clarke et al. 2000; Lu, Jan, and Jan 2000; Roy et al. 2000). Stem cells in the SVZ give rise to neuroblasts that migrate to the olfactory bulb and

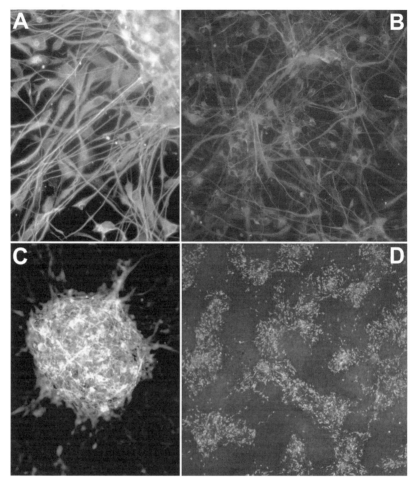

Figure 8. Human neural stem cells in culture. Photomicrographs are taken through the fluorescence microscope with different colors representing different proteins that are expressed by the cells. Some cells express multiple proteins while others express fewer. *(A)* Cells streaming out from a neurosphere (clump of cells in upper right corner). The green staining is nestin, a filamentous protein present in the cytoplasm of neural stem cells, while the red staining is Sox2, a transcription factor present in both embryonic and neural stem cells. These protein markers are commonly co-expressed. *(B)* Neural cell adhesion molecule staining (NCAM, red) and glial fibrillary acidic protein staining (GFAP, green) predominate in different subpopulations of cells and demonstrate the heterogeneity of the cultures. *(C)* Doublecortin (DCX, red), vimentin (green), and nestin (blue) staining in a neurosphere demonstrate the intimate commingling of the cells in a sphere as well as expression of multiple markers both in the same cells and in different cells. *(D)* These cells, grown from the neural retina, show staining common to brain neural stem cells (DCX, red) and staining found only in neural stem cells derived from the retina (recoverin, green). This shows that neural stem cells harvested from different parts of the nervous system may have certain intrinsic differences.

differentiate there (Gage 2002; Lu, Jan, and Jan 2000; Piper et al. 2000). In the developing cerebral wall of embryonic rodents, the cells at the ventricular surface generate their progeny by ACD (Miyata et al. 2004).

Human neural stem cells have been recovered from brain tissue removed from patients undergoing lobectomy (Johansson et al. 1999) and from donated fetal tissue (Flax et al. 1998; Svendsen, Caldwell, and Ostenfeld 1999; Tamaki et al. 2002; Vescovi et al. 1999). They can also be recovered from cadavers even as late as twenty hours after death (Palmer et al. 2001; P. Schwartz et al. 2003). These cells can proliferate for long periods in culture and can be grown in adherent monolayers or as neurospheres, depending on the conditions. They express immature neurodevelopmental markers including nestin (Frederiksen and McKay 1988; Lendahl, Zimmerman, and McKay 1990), Sox2 (Cai et al. 2002; Han et al. 1993; Zappone et al. 2000), and nucleostemin (Tsai and McKay 2002).

Neural stem cells in vitro show asymmetric localization of LGN (homolog of the *Drosophila* ACD determinant Pins; Fuja et al. 2004), but the consequences of this localization and the behavior of other ACD determinants have not been tested. These cells are generally considered to be derived from the SVZ, but in vivo the SVZ cells do not show any signs of ACD (Gleason et al. n.d.). However, we have recently shown that cells of the ependymal layer, which overlie the SVZ at the ventricular surface and are generally considered to be postmitotic in the adult, can be activated to proliferate by injury and that they show clear asymmetric localization of ACD markers. It therefore seems likely that the ependymal cells are true stem cells as defined by ACD and that they give rise to the SVZ cells, which proliferate further before they differentiate.

Other Mesenchymal and Tissue-Specific Stem Cells

In addition to bone marrow, other tissues contain stem cell populations that are capable of differentiating into mesenchymal derivatives and that are therefore called MSCs (Jiang et al. 2002; R. Schwartz et al. 2002). These cells have been found in periosteum, trabecular bone, adipose tissue, synovium, skeletal muscle, lung, and deciduous teeth, and most of them can differentiate into several tissue types.

Skin and Hair

Human skin consists of two distinct layers, each with different populations of stem cells. The lower 90 percent of skin, the dermis, provides most of the structural support and contains fibrous components (collagen and elastin) as well as ground substance, blood vessels, and nerves. Most of the cells found in dermis are fibroblasts, but multipotent stem cells have been isolated from the dermis of mice (Toma et al. 2001), and clones derived from these cells were shown to differentiate in vitro into neurons, glia, smooth muscle cells, and adipocytes (fat cells). The fact that these cells can produce both neural and mesodermal derivatives led to the suggestion that they may provide an easily accessible source of stem cells for therapeutic purposes.

The outer layer of skin, the epidermis, is continuous with the epithelial sheath of the hair follicles, and stem cells capable of producing both epidermis and hair follicles are located in a niche, called the bulge, at the base of each follicle in the outer root sheath (Amoh et al. 2004). These cells are identified as stem cells because of their slow cycling (shown by long-term retention of labeled precursors in DNA) and the presence of stem cell markers, including nestin. There may also be some stem cells, possibly with more limited potential than the bulge cells, between follicles (Ma, Yang, and Lee 2004). Genetically marked individual cells taken from the follicle bulge in a normal mouse, mixed with dermal cells, and grafted onto an immune-deficient mouse were able to form epidermis, outer root sheath, inner root sheath, hair shaft, and sebaceous gland (Morris et al. 2004), showing that they can produce all the cell types of the epidermal layer. Recently the bulge has been shown to also contain a distinct population of stem cells derived from the neural crest (Sieber-Blum and Grim 2004), which retain the ability to differentiate into known neural crest derivatives, including neurons, Schwann cells, smooth muscle cells, melanocytes, and chondrocytes.

The identification of stem cells in both dermis and epidermis marks a major advance in the effort to produce complete artificial skin, which would find enormous applications in treatment of burn injuries. The ability of bulge cells to regenerate hair structures also suggests that this kind of research could lead to treatments for hair loss (DeNoon 2004).

Stem Cells from Other Tissues

In addition to the examples cited above, several other organ systems have been investigated as possible sources of stem cells. These include intestinal mucosa (Marshman, Booth, and Potten 2002; Potten et al. 2003), liver (Xiao et al. 2004), lung (Kotton, Summer, and Fine 2004), heart (Hughes

2002), and skeletal muscle (Chen and Goldhamer 2003; Morgan and Partridge 2003). In all of these cases some troubling questions have arisen with respect to the origin of the stem cells. It is often very difficult to determine whether the stem cells are authentic components of the organ system where they are found or cells that have migrated from another source such as the bone marrow. These questions are under active investigation in many laboratories.

CONCLUSION

The human body is turning out to have many more stem cell populations than previously recognized, and many of them seem to have more developmental potential than expected. It seems very likely that in the near future we will see the discovery of methods to control the proliferation and differentiation of many kinds of stem cells, and technologies are already being developed for replacing the nuclei of stem cells with those of prospective patients so that immune rejection can be avoided. The enormous opportunities and challenges in the development of stem cell therapy are the subject of the following chapter.

REFERENCES

Altaba, A., P. Sanchez, and N. Dahmane.
    2002. Gli and hedgehog in cancer: Tumours, embryos and stem cells. Nat. Rev. Cancer 2:361–72.

Altman, J.
    1969. Autoradiographic and histological studies of postnatal neurogenesis. IV. Cell proliferation and migration in the anterior forebrain, with special reference to persisting neurogenesis in the olfactory bulb. J. Comp. Neurol. 137:433–57.

Amit, M., M. K. Carpenter, M. S. Inokuma, C. P. Chiu, C. P. Harris, M. A. Waknitz, J. Itskovitz-Eldor, and J. A. Thomson.
    2000. Clonally derived human embryonic stem cell lines maintain pluripotency and proliferative potential for prolonged periods of culture. Dev. Biol. 227:271–78.

Amoh, Y., L. Li, M. Yang, A. R. Moossa, K. Katsuoka, S. Penman, and R. M. Hoffman.
    2004. Nascent blood vessels in the skin arise from nestin-expressing hair-follicle cells. Proc. Natl. Acad. Sci. U.S.A. 101:13291–95.

Baroffio, A., E. Dupin, and N. M. Le Douarin.
    1991. Common precursors for neural and mesectodermal derivatives in the cephalic neural crest. Development 112:301–5.

Bodnar, M. S., J. J. Meneses, R. T. Rodriguez, and M. T. Firpo.
    2004. Propagation and maintenance of undifferentiated human embryonic stem cells. Stem Cells Dev. 13:243–53.

Brewer, G. J., and C. W. Cotman.
    1989. Survival and growth of hippocampal neurons in defined medium at low density: Advantages of a sandwich culture technique or low oxygen. Brain Res. 494:65–74.

Brustle, O., K. N. Jones, R. D. Learish, K. Karram, K. Choudhary, O. D. Wiestler, I. D. Duncan, and R. D. McKay.
    1999. Embryonic stem cell-derived glial precursors: A source of myelinating transplants. Science 285:754–56.

Cai, J., Y. Wu, T. Mirua, J. L. Pierce, M. T. Lucero, K. H. Albertine, G. J. Spangrude, and M. S. Rao.
    2002. Properties of a fetal multipotent neural stem cell (NEP cell). Dev. Biol. 251:221–40.

Carpenter, M. K., M. S. Inokuma, J. Denham, T. Mujtaba, C. P. Chiu, and M. S. Rao.
    2001. Enrichment of neurons and neural precursors from human embryonic stem cells. Exp. Neurol. 172:383–97.

Carpenter, M. K., E. S. Rosler, G. J. Fisk, R. Brandenberger, X. Ares, T. Miura, M. Lucero, and M. S. Rao.
    2004. Properties of four human embryonic stem cell lines maintained in a feeder-free culture system. Dev. Dyn. 229:243–58.

Carpenter, M. K., E. Rosler, and M. S. Rao.
    2003. Characterization and differentiation of human embryonic stem cells. Cloning Stem Cells 5:79–88.

Chen, J. C., and D. J. Goldhamer.
    2003. Skeletal muscle stem cells. Reprod. Biol. Endocrinol. 1:101.

Chenn, A., and S. K. McConnell.
    1995. Cleavage orientation and the asymmetric inheritance of Notch1 immunoreactivity in mammalian neurogenesis. Cell 82:631–41.

Chiasson, B. J., V. Tropepe, C. M. Morshead, and D. van der Kooy.
    1999. Adult mammalian forebrain ependymal and subependymal cells demonstrate proliferative potential, but only subependymal cells have neural stem cell characteristics. J. Neurosci. 19:4462–71.

Clarke, D. L., C. B. Johansson, J. Wilbertz, B. Veress, E. Nilsson, H. Karlstrom, U. Lendahl, and J. Frisen.
    2000. Generalized potential of adult neural stem cells. Science 288:1660–63.

Conboy, I. M., and T. A. Rando.
    2002. The regulation of Notch signaling controls satellite cell activation and cell fate determination in postnatal myogenesis. Dev. Cell 3:397–409.

Cowan, C. A., I. Klimanskaya, J. McMahon, J. Atienza, J. Witmyer, J. P. Zucker, S. Wang, C. C. Morton, A. P. McMahon, D. Powers, and D. A. Melton.

2004. Derivation of embryonic stem-cell lines from human blastocysts. N. Engl. J. Med. 350:1353–56.

Dekel, I., Y. Magal, S. Pearson-White, C. P. Emerson, and M. Shani.
1992. Conditional conversion of ES cells to skeletal muscle by an exogenous MyoD1 gene. New Biol. 4:217–24.

Dennis, J. E., and A. I. Caplan.
2003. Bone marrow mesenchymal stem cells. In: S. Sell, ed. Stem Cells Handbook, 107–18. Totowa, NJ: Humana Press.

DeNoon, D.
2004. Hair cloning nears reality as baldness cure: Hair multiplication puts new face on hair restoration. WebMD Health. Nov. 4.

Doetsch, F.
2003. A niche for adult neural stem cells. Curr. Opin. Genet. Dev. 13:543–50.

Doetsch, F., I. Caille, D. A. Lim, J. M. Garcia-Verdugo, and A. Alvarez-Buylla.
1999. Subventricular zone astrocytes are neural stem cells in the adult mammalian brain. Cell 97:703–16.

Eriksson, P. S., E. Perfilieva, T. Bjork-Eriksson, A. M. Alborn, C. Nordborg, D. A. Peterson, and F. H. Gage.
1998. Neurogenesis in the adult human hippocampus. Nat. Med. 4:1313–17.

Fang, C. M., and Y. H. Xu.
2001. Down-regulated expression of atypical PKC-binding domain deleted asip isoforms in human hepatocellular carcinomas. Cell Res. 11:223–29.

Flax, J. D., S. Aurora, C. Yang, C. Simonin, A. M. Wills, L. L. Billinghurst, M. Jendoubi, R. L. Sidman, J. H. Wolfe, S. U. Kim, and E. Y. Snyder.
1998. Engraftable human neural stem cells respond to developmental cues, replace neurons, and express foreign genes. Nat. Biotechnol. 16: 1033–39.

Frederiksen, K., and R. D. McKay.
1988. Proliferation and differentiation of rat neuroepithelial precursor cells in vivo. J. Neurosci. 8:1144–51.

Fuchs, E., T. Tumbar, and G. Guasch.
2004. Socializing with the neighbors: Stem cells and their niche. Cell 116 (6): 769–78.

Fuja, T. J., P. H. Schwartz, D. Darcy, and P. J. Bryant.
2004. Asymmetric localization of LGN but not AGS3, two homologs of Drosophila pins, in dividing human neural progenitor cells. J. Neurosci. Res. 75:782–93.

Gage, F. H.
1998. Stem cells of the central nervous system. Curr. Opin. Neurobiol. 8:671–76.
2002. Neurogenesis in the adult brain. J. Neurosci. 22:612–13.

Garcia-Verdugo, J. M., F. Doetsch, H. Wichterle, D. A. Lim, and A. Alvarez-Buylla.

1998. Architecture and cell types of the adult subventricular zone: In search of the stem cells. J. Neurobiol. 36:234–48.

Gould, E., A. J. Reeves, M. S. Graziano, and C. G. Gross.
1999. Neurogenesis in the neocortex of adult primates. Science 286:548–52.

Gussoni, E., Y. Soneoka, C. D. Strickland, E. A., Buzney, M. K. Khan, A. F. Flint, L. M. Kunkel, and R. C. Mulligan.
1999. Dystrophin expression in the mdx mouse restored by stem cell transplantation. Nature 401:390–94.

Han, M., A. Golden, Y. Han, and P. W. Sternberg.
1993. C. elegans lin-45 raf gene participates in let-60 ras-stimulated vulval differentiation. Nature 363:133–40.

Hauwel, M., E. Furon, and P. Gasque.
2005. Molecular and cellular insights into the coxsackie-adenovirus receptor: Role in cellular interactions in the stem cell niche. Brain Res. Rev. 48: 265–72.

He, J. Q., Y. Ma, Y. Lee, J. A. Thomson, and T. J. Kamp.
2003. Human embryonic stem cells develop into multiple types of cardiac myocytes: Action potential characterization. Circ. Res. 93:32–39.

Hermann, A., R. Gastl, S. Liebau, M. O. Popa, J. Fiedler, B. O. Boehm, M. Maisel, H. Lerche, J. Schwarz, R. Brenner, and A. Storch.
2004. Efficient generation of neural stem cell-like cells from adult human bone marrow stromal cells. J. Cell Sci. 117:4411–22.

Hughes, S.
2002. Cardiac stem cells. J. Pathol. 197:468–78.

Huttmann, A., C. L. Li, and U. Duhrsen.
2003. Bone marrow-derived stem cells and "plasticity." Ann. Hematol. 82:599–604.

Jiang, Y., B. N. Jahagirdar, R. L. Reinhardt, R. E. Schwartz, C. D. Keene, X. R. Ortiz-Gonzalez, M. Reyes, T. Lenvik, T. Lund, M. Blackstad, J. Du, S. Aldrich, A. Lisberg, W. C. Low, D. A. Largaespada, and C. M. Verfaillie.
2002. Pluripotency of mesenchymal stem cells derived from adult marrow. Nature 418:41–49.

Johansson, C. B., M. Svensson, L. Wallstedt, A. M. Janson, and J. Frisen.
1999. Neural stem cells in the adult human brain. Exp. Cell Res. 253:733–36.

Justice, N. J., and Y. N. Jan.
2002. Variations on the Notch pathway in neural development. Curr. Opin. Neurobiol. 12:64–70.

Kim, J. H., J. M. Auerbach, J. A. Rodriguez-Gomez, I. Velasco, D. Gavin, N. Lumelsky, S. H. Lee, J. Nguyen, R. Sanchez-Pernaute, K. Bankiewicz, and R. McKay.
2002. Dopamine neurons derived from embryonic stem cells function in an animal model of Parkinson's disease. Nature 418:50–56.

Klug, M. G., M. H. Soonpaa, G. Y. Koh, and L. J. Field.
  1996. Genetically selected cardiomyocytes from differentiating embronic stem cells form stable intracardiac grafts. J. Clin. Invest. 98:216–24.

Kotton, D. N., R. Summer, and A. Fine.
  2004. Lung stem cells: New paradigms. Exp. Hematol. 32:340–43.

Krause, H. M., and W. J. Gehring.
  1989. Stage-specific phosphorylation of the fushi tarazu protein during Drosophila development. EMBO J. 8:1197–1204.

Lagasse, E., H. Connors, M. Al Dhalimy, M. Reitsma, M. Dohse, L. Osborne, X. Wang, M. Finegold, I. L. Weissman, and M. Grompe.
  2000. Purified hematopoietic stem cells can differentiate into hepatocytes in vivo. Nat. Med. 6:1229–34.

Lanza, R., M. A. Moore, T. Wakayama, A. C. Perry, J. H. Shieh, J. Hendrikx, A. Leri, S. Chimenti, A. Monsen, D. Nurzynska, M. D. West, J. Kajstura, and P. Anversa.
  2004. Regeneration of the infarcted heart with stem cells derived by nuclear transplantation. Circ. Res. 94:820–27.

Le Douarin, N. M., and E. Dupin.
  2003. Multipotentiality of the neural crest. Curr. Opin. Genet. Dev. 13:529–36.

Lendahl, U., L. B. Zimmerman, and R. D. McKay.
  1990. CNS stem cells express a new class of intermediate filament protein. Cell 60:585–95.

Lu, B., L. Jan, and Y. N. Jan.
  2000. Control of cell divisions in the nervous system: Symmetry and asymmetry. Annu. Rev. Neurosci. 23:531–56.

Ma, D. R., E. N. Yang, and S. T. Lee.
  2004. A review: The location, molecular characterisation and multipotency of hair follicle epidermal stem cells. Ann. Acad. Med. Singapore 33:784–88.

Marshman, E., C. Booth, and C. S. Potten.
  2002. The intestinal epithelial stem cell. BioEssays 24:91–98.

Mathur, A., and J. F. Martin.
  2004. Stem cells and repair of the heart. Lancet 364:183–92.

Matsuzaki, F.
  2000. Asymmetric division of Drosophila neural stem cells: A basis for neural diversity. Curr. Opin. Neurobiol. 10:38–44.

McKay, R.
  1997. Stem cells in the central nervous system. Science 276:66–71.

Mezey, E., S. Key, G. Vogelsang, I. Szalayova, G. D. Lange, and B. Crain.
  2003. Transplanted bone marrow generates new neurons in human brains. Proc. Natl. Acad. Sci. U.S.A. 100:1364–69.

Miyata, T., A. Kawaguchi, K. Saito, M. Kawano, T. Muto, and M. Ogawa.
2004. Asymmetric production of surface-dividing and non-surface-dividing cortical progenitor cells. Development 131:3133–45.

Mochizuki, N., G. Cho, B. Wen, and P. A. Insel.
1996. Identification and cDNA cloning of a novel human mosaic protein, LGN, based on interaction with G alpha i2. Gene 181:39–43.

Morgan, J. E., and T. A. Partridge.
2003. Muscle satellite cells. Int. J. Biochem. Cell Biol. 35:1151–56.

Morris, R. J., Y. Liu, L. Marles, Z. Yang, C. Trempus, S. Li, J. S. Lin, J. A. Sawicki, and G. Cotsarelis.
2004. Capturing and profiling adult hair follicle stem cells. Nat. Biotechnol. 22:411–17.

Morshead, C. M., B. A. Reynolds, C. G. Craig, M. W. McBurney, W. A. Staines, D. Morassutti, S. Weiss, and D. van der Kooy.
1994. Neural stem cells in the adult mammalian forebrain: A relatively quiescent subpopulation of subependymal cells. Neuron 13:1071–82.

Nistor, G. I., M. O. Totoiu, N. Haque, M. K. Carpenter, and, H. S. Keirstead.
2005. Human embryonic stem cells differentiate into oligodendrocytes in high purity and myelinate after spinal cord transplantation. Glia 49: 385–96.

Odorico, J. S., D. S. Kaufman, and J. A. Thomson.
2001. Multilineage differentiation from human embryonic stem cell lines. Stem Cells 19:193–204.

Orlic, D., J. Kajstura, S. Chimenti, I. Jakoniuk, S. M. Anderson, B. Li, J. Pickel, R. McKay, B. Nadal-Ginard, D. M. Bodine, A. Leri, and P. Anversa.
2001. Bone marrow cells regenerate infarcted myocardium. Nature 410:701–5.

Palmer, T. D., P. H. Schwartz, P. Taupin, B. Kaspar, S. A. Stein, and F. H. Gage.
2001. Cell culture: Progenitor cells from human brain after death. Nature 411:42–43.

Palmer, T. D., J. Takahashi, and F. H. Gage.
1997. The adult rat hippocampus contains primordial neural stem cells. Mol. Cell Neurosci. 8:389–404.

Perrier, A. L., V. Tabar, T. Barberi, M. E. Rubio, J. Bruses, N. Topf, N. L. Harrison, and L. Studer.
2004. Derivation of midbrain dopamine neurons from human embryonic stem cells. Proc. Natl. Acad. Sci. U.S.A. 101:12543–48.

Petersen, B. E., W. C. Bowen, K. D. Patrene, W. M. Mars, A. K. Sullivan, N. Murase, S. S. Boggs, J. S. Greenberger, and J. P. Goff.
1999. Bone marrow as a potential source of hepatic oval cells. Science 284:1168–70.

Piper, D. R., T. Mujtaba, M. S. Rao, and M. T. Lucero.
2000. Immunocytochemical and physiological characterization of a population of cultured human neural precursors. J. Neurophysiol. 84:534–48.

Pittenger, M. F., A. M. Mackay, S. C. Beck, R. K. Jaiswal, R. Douglas, J. D. Mosca, M. A. Moorman, D. W. Simonetti, S. Craig, and D. R. Marshak.
1999. Multilineage potential of adult human mesenchymal stem cells. Science 284:143–47.

Ponting, I., Y. Zhao, and W. F. Anderson.
2003. Hematopoietic stem cells: Identification, characterization, and assays. In: S. Sell, ed. Stem Cells Handbook, 155–62. Totowa, NJ: Humana Press.

Potten, C. S.
1997. Stem cells. San Diego: Academic Press.

Potten, C. S., C. Booth, G. L. Tudor, D. Booth, G. Brady, P. Hurley, G. Ashton, R. Clarke, S. Sakakibara, and H. Okano.
2003. Identification of a putative intestinal stem cell and early lineage marker: Musashi-1. Differentiation 71:28–41.

Rambhatla, L., C. P. Chiu, P. Kundu, Y. Peng, and M. K. Carpenter.
2003. Generation of hepatocyte-like cells from human embryonic stem cells. Cell Transplant. 12:1–11.

Reubinoff, B. E., P. Itsykson, T. Turetsky, M. F. Pera, E. Reinhartz, A. Itzik, and T. Ben Hur.
2001. Neural progenitors from human embryonic stem cells. Nat. Biotechnol. 19:1134–40.

Reynolds, B. A., W. Tetzlaff, and S. Weiss.
1992. A multipotent EGF-responsive striatal embryonic progenitor cell produces neurons and astrocytes. J. Neurosci. 12:4565–74.

Reynolds, B. A., and S. Weiss.
1996. Clonal and population analyses demonstrate that an EGF-responsive mammalian embryonic CNS precursor is a stem cell. Dev. Biol. 175: 1–13.

Rosler, E. S., G. J. Fisk, X. Ares, J. Irving, T. Miura, M. S. Rao, and M. K. Carpenter.
2004. Long-term culture of human embryonic stem cells in feeder-free conditions. Dev. Dyn. 229:259–74.

Roy, N. S., A. Benraiss, S. Wang, R. A. Fraser, R. Goodman, W. T. Couldwell, M. Nedergaard, A. Kawaguchi, H. Okano, and S. A. Goldman.
2000. Promoter-targeted selection and isolation of neural progenitor cells from the adult human ventricular zone. J. Neurosci. Res. 59:321–31.

Schofield, R.
1983. The stem cell system. Biomed. Pharmacother. 37:375–80.

Schuldiner, M., R. Eiges, A. Eden, O. Yanuka, J. Itskovitz-Eldor, R. S. Goldstein, and N. Benvenisty.
2001. Induced neuronal differentiation of human embryonic stem cells. Brain Res. 913:201–5.

Schwartz, P. H., P. J. Bryant, T. J. Fuja, H. Su, D. K. O'Dowd, and H. Klassen.
2003. Isolation and characterization of neural progenitor cells from postmortem human cortex. J. Neurosci. Res. 74:838–51.

Schwartz, R. E., M. Reyes, L. Koodie, Y. Jiang, M. Blackstad, T. Lund, T. Lenvik, S. Johnson, W. S. Hu, and C. M. Verfaillie.
2002. Multipotent adult progenitor cells from bone marrow differentiate into functional hepatocyte-like cells. J. Clin. Invest. 109 (10): 1291–1302.

Sell, S.
2003. Stem cells: What are they? Where do they come from? Why are they here? When do they go wrong? Where are they going? In: S. Sell, ed. Stem Cells Handbook, 1–18. Totowa, NJ: Humana Press.

Shen, Q., W. Zhong, Y. N. Jan, and S. Temple.
2002. Asymmetric Numb distribution is critical for asymmetric cell division of mouse cerebral cortical stem cells and neuroblasts. Development 129:4843–53.

Sherley, J. L.
2002. Asymmetric cell kinetics genes: The key to expansion of adult stem cells in culture. Sci. World J. 2:1906–21.

Shufaro, Y., and B. E. Reubinoff.
2004. Therapeutic applications of embryonic stem cells. Best. Pract. Res. Clin. Obstet. Gynaecol. 18:909–27.

Sieber-Blum, M., and M. Grim.
2004. The adult hair follicle: Cradle for pluripotent neural crest stem cells. Birth Defects Res. C. Embryo. Today 72:162–72.

Sieber-Blum, M., M. Grim, Y. F. Hu, and V. Szeder.
2004. Pluripotent neural crest stem cells in the adult hair follicle. Dev. Dyn. 231:258–69.

Svendsen, C. N., M. A. Caldwell, and T. Ostenfeld.
1999. Human neural stem cells: Isolation, expansion and transplantation. Brain Pathol. 9:499–513.

Tabar, V., G. Panagiotakos, E. D. Greenberg, B. K. Chan, M. Sadelain, P. H. Gutin, and L. Studer.
2005. Migration and differentiation of neural precursors derived from human embryonic stem cells in the rat brain. Nat. Biotech. 23:601–6.

Takano, H., H. Ema, K. Sudo, and H. Nakauchi.
2004. Asymmetric division and lineage commitment at the level of hematopoietic stem cells: Inference from differentiation in daughter cell and granddaughter cell pairs. J. Exp. Med. 199:295–302.

Tamaki, S., K. Eckert, D. He, R. Sutton, M. Doshe, G. Jain, R. Tushinski, M. Reitsma, B. Harris, A. Tsukamoto, F. Gage, I. Weissman, and N. Uchida.
2002. Engraftment of sorted/expanded human central nervous system stem cells from fetal brain. J. Neurosci. Res. 69:976–86.

Temple, S.
2001. The development of neural stem cells. Nature 414:12–117.

Theise, N. D., M. Nimmakayalu, R. Gardner, P. B. Illei, G. Morgan, L. Teperman, O. Henegariu, and D. S. Krause.
2000. Liver from bone marrow in humans. Hepatology 32:11–16.

Thiele, J., E. Varus, C. Wickenhauser, H. M. Kvasnicka, K. Metz, U. W. Schaefer, and D. W. Beelen.
2002. [Chimerism of cardiomyocytes and endothelial cells after allogeneic bone marrow transplantation in chronic myeloid leukemia: An autopsy study]. Pathologe 23:405–10.

Thomson, J. A., J. Itskovitz-Eldor, S. S. Shapiro, M. A. Waknitz, J. J. Swiergiel, V. S. Marshall, and J. M. Jones.
1998. Embryonic stem cell lines derived from human blastocysts. Science 282:1145–47.

Toma, J. G., M. Akhavan, K. J. L. Fernandes, F. Barnabe-Heider, A. Sadikot, D. R. Kaplan, and F. D. Miller.
2001. Isolation of multipotent adult stem cells from the dermis of mammalian skin. Nat. Cell. Biol. 3:778–84.

Trounson, A.
2004. Stem cells, plasticity and cancer: Uncomfortable bed fellows. Development 131:2763–68.

Tsai, R. Y., and R. D. McKay.
2002. A nucleolar mechanism controlling cell proliferation in stem cells and cancer cells. Genes Dev. 16:2991–3003.

Uchida, N., D. W. Buck, D. He, M. J. Reitsma, M. Masek, T. V. Phan, A. S. Tsukamoto, F. H. Gage, and I. L. Weissman.
2000. Direct isolation of human central nervous system stem cells. Proc. Natl. Acad. Sci. U.S.A. 97:14720–25.

Venters, S. J., and C. P. Ordahl.
2005. Asymmetric cell divisions are concentrated in the dermomyotome dorsomedial lip during epaxial primary myotome morphogenesis. Anat. Embryol. 209 (6): 449–60.

Vescovi, A. L., E. A. Parati, A. Gritti, P. Poulin, M. Ferrario, E. Wanke, P. Frolichsthal-Schoeller, L. Cova, M. Arcellana-Panlilio, A. Colombo, and R. Galli.
1999. Isolation and cloning of multipotential stem cells from the embryonic human CNS and establishment of transplantable human neural stem cell lines by epigenetic stimulation. Exp. Neurol. 156:71–83.

Wang, X., H. Willenbring, Y. Akkari, Y. Torimaru, M. Foster, M. Al Dhalimy, E. Lagasse, M. Finegold, S. Olson, and M. Grompe.
2003. Cell fusion is the principal source of bone-marrow-derived hepatocytes. Nature 422:897–901.

Wernig, M., F. Benninger, T. Schmandt, M. Rade, K. L. Tucker, H. Bussow, H. Beck, and O. Brustle.
2004. Functional integration of embryonic stem cell-derived neurons in vivo. J. Neurosci. 24:5258–68.

Xiao, J. C., X. L. Jin, P. Ruck, A. Adam, and E. Kaiserling.
2004. Hepatic progenitor cells in human liver cirrhosis: Immunohistochemical, electron microscopic and immunofluorence confocal microscopic findings. World J. Gastroenterol. 10:1208–11.

Xu, C., M. S. Inokuma, J. Denham, K. Golds, P. Kundu, J. D. Gold, and M. K. Carpenter.
2001. Feeder-free growth of undifferentiated human embryonic stem cells. Nat. Biotechnol. 19:971–74.

Xu, C., S. Police, N. Rao, and, M. K. Carpenter.
2002. Characterization and enrichment of cardiomyocytes derived from human embryonic stem cells. Circ. Res. 91:501–8.

Zappone, M. V., R. Galli, R. Catena, N. Meani, S. De Biasi, E. Mattei, C. Tiveron, A. L. Vescovi, R. Lovell-Badge, S. Ottolenghi, and, S. K. Nicolis.
2000. Sox2 regulatory sequences direct expression of a (beta)-geo transgene to telencephalic neural stem cells and precursors of the mouse embryo, revealing regionalization of gene expression in CNS stem cells. Development 127:2367–82.

Zhan, X., G. Dravid, Z. Ye, H. Hammond, M. Shamblott, J. Gearhart, and L. Cheng.
2004. Functional antigen-presenting leucocytes derived from human embryonic stem cells in vitro. Lancet 364:163–71.

Zhang, R. L., Z. G. Zhang, L. Zhang, and M. Chopp.
2001. Proliferation and differentiation of progenitor cells in the cortex and the subventricular zone in the adult rat after focal cerebral ischemia. Neuroscience 105:33–41.

Zhong, W., J. N. Feder, M. M. Jiang, L. Y. Jan, and Y. N. Jan.
1996. Asymmetric localization of a mammalian Numb homolog during mouse cortical neurogenesis. Neuron 17:43–53.

Zhong, W., M. M. Jiang, G. Weinmaster, L. Y. Jan, and Y. N.
1997. Differential expression of mammalian Numb, Numblike and Notch1 suggests distinct roles during mouse cortical neurogenesis. Development 124:1887–97.

CHAPTER 2

Therapeutic Uses of Stem Cells

Philip H. Schwartz and Peter J. Bryant

It has been estimated that over 100 million patients in the United States might benefit from stem cell–based therapies. The most numerous of these patients are those affected by cardiovascular disease (79.4 million, American Heart Association 2007), autoimmune diseases (14.7 to 23.5 million, National Institute of Allergy and Infectious Diseases 2005), type 1 and type 2 diabetes (20.8 million, American Diabetes Association 2007), osteoporosis (10 million, National Institute of Arthritis and Musculoskeletal and Skin Diseases 2007), cancer (10.5 million, National Cancer Institute 2006), Alzheimer's disease (4.5 million, Alzheimer's Association 2005), and Parkinson's disease (1.5 million, American Parkinson's Disease Association 2003).

Stem cell therapy, using bone marrow, umbilical cord blood, or peripheral blood stem cells, has been critically important in the clinical treatment of several disorders of the blood and immune systems, including lymphomas and leukemias, raising hopes that similar treatments for other organ systems may be developed using stem cells from embryos or solid adult tissues. In the case of lymphomas and leukemias, the transplanted stem cells help the patient by directly differentiating into the expected blood or immune cell type and restoring the missing function at the cellular level. This, too, has been the hope for stem cell therapy used for diseased or damaged solid tissues. However, studies on model systems have revealed a surprisingly large number of other ways in which stem cell therapy may provide benefits. Transplanted stem cells can provoke the multiplication and function of the host stem cells, prevent further loss and damage of host tissues, or stimulate the production of new blood vessels that can help restore host tissues. The transplanted cells presumably produce these effects by producing growth factors and other products that are locally active. Transplanted stem cells can also fuse with host cells, and this can help repair damage even if the transplanted cells are not completely transformed into the target tissue type.

CURRENT THERAPEUTIC APPLICATIONS

Blood and Immune System Disorders

Transplantation of bone marrow, containing hematopoietic stem cells (HSCs), or of purified cell fractions from bone marrow has been used for over three decades in the treatment of disorders of the blood cell production system. Children with severe combined immune deficiency have been successfully treated by bone marrow transplantation since 1968 (Baird 2003). Leukemia patients have been successfully treated with radio- and chemotherapy to destroy the bone marrow (myeloablation) and cancer cells, followed by rescue with bone marrow transplants from human leukocyte antigen (HLA)-identical twins or siblings or HLA-matched donors (Baird 2003). For lymphoma and leukemia, the patient's own bone marrow may be harvested in advance when the disease is in remission, cleared of undesirable cells (residual malignant cells and cells that could mediate a graft-versus-host immune reaction), and frozen so that it can subsequently be used to restore the patient's hematopoietic system after myeloablation. More recently, peripheral blood (after treatment of the donor with cytokines to mobilize stem cells) has been found to be a better source of stem cells to restore hematopoiesis (Baird 2003). Umbilical cord blood (UCB) can also be used and has several advantages over bone marrow as a source of HSCs, especially in pediatric patients (Lewis 2002). It is less likely to cause problems with graft-versus-host disease, it contains more primitive stem cells, and the stem cells appear to have greater proliferative potential than bone marrow cells. In addition, UCB stem cells implant and function as stem cells at lower cell doses than bone marrow or peripheral blood cells (Lewis 2002). However, engrafting is often delayed (possibly due to lower cell numbers), and reconstitution of the immune system, which is critical for host recovery, can be more delayed than is the case for bone marrow (Lewis 2002).

Metabolic Diseases

Another group of diseases being treated with HSC transplantation is the lysosomal storage disorders, including the mucopolysaccharidoses such as Hurler's syndrome. These diseases involve the harmful accumulation of specific cell components, due to the absence or inactivity of a specific enzyme normally involved in their degradation. In these cases, stem cell therapy would function primarily for enzyme replacement, by providing cells containing an active form of the missing or defective enzyme. Since disease progression may lead to extensive damage, early diagnosis and treatment are essential (Malatack et al. 2003). At present, HSC transplantation is effective primarily for soft tissue, non–central nervous system organs such as spleen and liver, with only limited effectiveness for bone and cartilage and little to no effectiveness for the central nervous system (Malatack et al. 2003).

EXPERIMENTAL THERAPEUTIC APPLICATIONS

Multiple Sclerosis (MS)

This is a debilitating neurological disease in which chronic inflammation of the central nervous system leads to multiple impairments of motor, sensory, and cognitive functions. It affects about a million people worldwide, about two hundred thousand of them in the United States. The fundamental feature of the disorder is that the individual's own immune system attacks and destroys the myelin sheath that normally surrounds nerve fibers and provides them with the equivalent of electrical insulation. Some of the destroyed myelin regenerates spontaneously, although it is not clear exactly which cell type is responsible for producing this myelin. Current treatments mainly use the immunomodulator beta-interferon to slow the progression of the disease.

Two different manipulations of stem cell populations are being tested as potential treatments for MS. First, since the disease results mainly from the development of a population of immune cells that attack the myelin sheaths of neurons, the replacement of the stem cell population generating these immune cells is a logical goal. In fact, the possibility of this kind of treatment was first recognized when some MS patients being treated by transplants of blood stem cells for other diseases showed remission of their MS symptoms. In a clinical trial of hematopoietic stem cell (HSC) transplantation for MS, twenty out of twenty-six patients appeared to stabilize (Nash et al., 2003). These trials included a combination of total body irradiation and chemotherapy followed by peripheral blood stem cell transplantation. About 250 patients are currently in phase 1 and phase 2 open clinical trials (Sykes and Nikolic 2005).

Soon after their discovery, neural stem cells (NSCs) were recognized as having tremendous potential for the cell-based repair of neurological damage from central nervous system injury and stroke, as well as for therapy of otherwise incurable diseases such as Huntington's disease and amyotrophic lateral sclerosis (Rice et al. 2003). However, it seems likely that the first applications will be for therapy of neurological diseases that do not require the establishment of new neuronal circuitry, notably MS (Furlan et al. 2003; Pluchino, Furlan, et al. 2004; Pluchino, Quattrini, et al. 2003), Parkinson's disease (Drucker-Colin and Verdugo-Diaz 2004), and metabolic diseases. Thus NSC therapy could be used to repair the demyelination caused by the immune attack. NSCs support the production of neurons and glia in parts of the normal brain throughout adulthood. They can be isolated from either fetal or adult brains, expanded extensively, and maintained safely in a chemically defined medium; they can be directed into a neuronal fate or an astrocyte fate by treatment with different growth factors; and they can be safely frozen and thawed, thus eliminating the need for continuous maintenance (Nunes et al. 2003; Schwartz et al. 2003; Vescovi et al. 1999). Their ability to migrate over long distances in the body and to apparently home in on diseased areas also makes them uniquely suitable for cell therapy of diseases, including MS, that are "multifocal" (affecting many locations in the body) (Imitola et al. 2004).

In a mouse model of MS (experimental autoimmune encephalomyelitis), NSCs implanted into the brain survived well and could home in on the demyelinated region, differentiate into oligodendrocytes, stimulate the increased production of host oligodendrocytes, and remyelinate the damaged fibers. They also reduced astrogliosis (excess production of astrocytes and the buildup of an astroglial scar), further demyelination, and axon loss (Pluchino, Quattrini, et al. 2003). These cells were equally effective if administered via the circulation, after which they passed through the blood-brain barrier and entered the brain. Many of the treated mice were completely cured of the disease, and the cells did not produce tumors.

Embryonic stem cells (ESCs) are also an attractive option for treatment of demyelinating diseases. When transplanted into rodents suffering from demyelinating disease, they can differentiate into glial cells and remyelinate affected axons (Brustle et al. 1999; Liu et al. 2000; McDonald et al. 1999). However, these cells also produce tumors called teratomas (Brustle et al. 1997), so the controls over their differentiation will have to be analyzed more thoroughly before they can be seriously considered for use in stem cell therapy. It has already been shown that ESCs can be induced to differentiate into oligodendrocyte precursors and that these can be used to promote myelination of axons in the shiverer mouse (Nistor et al. 2005), which suffers from defective myelination.

The remarkable ability of stem cells to home in on diseased areas appears to be a response to the inflammation at the disease site. Inflammation involves the production of a well-characterized set of molecules, including proteins that function in adhesion between cells (e.g., integrins), proteins that act as signals between cells to attract them to each other and to activate them in various ways (chemokines and cytokines), and specific receptors for these proteins (Cottler-Fox et al. 2003; Lapidot and Petit 2002). An intriguing discovery regarding the mechanism was that two proteins (CD44 and Very Late Antigen-4), shown to be required for NSCs to home in on inflamed regions, are the same proteins that attracted the inflammatory lymphocytes to the site in the first place (Pluchino, Furlan, et al. 2004).

POTENTIAL THERAPEUTIC APPLICATIONS

Parkinson's Disease

Parkinson's disease, which is marked by tremors and rigidity, affects about 1 million Americans. The disease is caused by the death of dopamine-secreting cells in the brain and is a prime candidate for cell-based therapies. In animal studies, treatment with glial cell line–derived neurotrophic factor (GDNF) promoted survival and growth of dopaminergic neurons (Burke 2004), and intracerebral infusion of this factor showed early signs of promise in clinical trials on human patients (Grondin et al. 2003). However, these trials were stopped when the improvements were attributed to a placebo effect and further animal experiments with higher doses revealed safety issues (Pollack 2004). Implants of fetal cells also showed early promise but were ultimately attributed to placebo effects (Roitberg et al. 2004).

The conversion of neural progenitor cells to dopaminergic neurons can be promoted by treatment in vitro with several neurotrophic factors, including GDNF (Riaz et al. 2004), and ESCs can be genetically engineered to show the dopaminergic phenotype (Kim 2004), suggesting that modified stem cells could be used in cell therapy for Parkinson's disease.

But, as with other proposed stem-cell therapies, an autologous source of cells that could be engineered or transdifferentiated to provide therapeutic functions might be preferable to heterologous cells that would require immunosuppression. Both retinal and iris pigmented epithelial cells, which can be isolated from the patient with different degrees of invasive surgery, produce neurotrophic factors including GDNF and are being investigated for use in cell-based therapy for Parkinson's disease (Arnhold, Semkova, et al. 2004b).

Spinal Cord Injury

When implanted into a diseased or injured brain, NSCs can migrate great distances to the site of disease or injury (Yip et al. 2003). Once there, the cells presumably respond to local cues and differentiate into appropriate cell types and integrate into the tissue. Recent studies have also suggested that these implanted cells can also elicit protective or regenerative responses from the local cells. The ability of NSCs to migrate within the central nervous system has also suggested that they may be used as vectors for gene therapy in cases where the gene product is diffusible and can therefore benefit other cells in the tissue: for example, they could be used for the delivery of therapeutic proteins and growth factors to promote axonal repair after spinal cord injury (Lu et al. 2003). Studies have also suggested that ESCs, induced to differentiate into oligodendroglia precursors, may have therapeutic effects in the treatment of spinal cord injury by contributing, directly or indirectly, to remyelination (Keirstead et al. 2005).

Retinal Degeneration

Retinal degenerative diseases, including retinitis pigmentosa and age-related macular degeneration, represent a major source of untreatable visual loss. Currently available therapies are not very effective and do not replace lost neurons. Work on animal systems has shown that transplanted NSCs can migrate into a diseased retina and that they can differentiate in a manner appropriate to their location (Takahashi et al. 1998; Young et al. 2000). Stem cells specific to the retina (retinal progenitor cells) have been isolated from the retina of mice (Shatos et al. 2001), human abortuses (Kelley et al. 1995; Yang et al. 2002), and post mortem premature infants (Klassen et al. 2004). In the latter case, viable progenitor cells were cultured from the post mortem retina and showed a gene expression profile consistent with their being immature neuroepithelial cells. These results suggest that retinal stem cells could be collected and could provide the underpinnings for a strategy aimed at treating retinal degenerative diseases.

Type 1 Diabetes

About one in every four hundred to five hundred children and adolescents in the United States (eight hundred thousand individuals) suffers from type 1 (insulin-dependent or juvenile onset) diabetes, in which the insulin-producing cells of the pancreas are lost and the body does not produce any insulin. A much larger number of people have type 2 (insulin-resistant) diabetes, in which cells of the body fail to respond to insulin. Some type 1 diabetes patients have received pancreas transplants, and many of these patients' diabetes symptoms disappear. However, the demand for transplants far outweighs the availability of donors, and patients who do get transplants must take powerful immune suppression medication to prevent rejection of the transplanted pancreas. Other therapies have relied on injection of the pancreatic islet cells, the cells that actually produce pancreatic insulin, but these cell-based therapies also rely on available donors (typically two per recipient) and lifelong immune suppression.

Research on potential new cell-based therapies for the treatment of diabetes has recently begun using ESCs rather than differentiated islet cells (Berna et al. 2001; Lechner and Habener 2003; Miyamoto 2001). This approach has the advantage that great numbers of these cells can be grown in the laboratory, reducing the number of tissue donors needed and potentially increasing the availability of the treatment to many more patients. Although scientists have been successful in getting the stem cells to differentiate into functional cells capable of producing insulin, it has been difficult to direct them to react appropriately to the body's signaling mechanisms that dictate the level of insulin production. In addition, some investigators have been using genetic engineering approaches to coerce adult stem cells into producing insulin. Once the cells do so, however, they are much less inclined to propagate, suggesting that a balance between proliferation and differentiation must be achieved before the technique can have general clinical applicability.

Brain Tumors

NSCs have a remarkable ability to migrate through the body and through normal tissues to accumulate in various types of tumors, both neural and non-neural (Ehtesham et al. 2002). This provides a potential avenue to developing radically new types of cancer treatment, especially for tumors that infiltrate the brain so extensively that they cannot be effectively removed by surgery or chemotherapy. In such cases, it may be possible to use the homing ability of NSCs to deliver chemotherapeutic agents accurately and exclusively to the tumor cells.

In studies on an experimentally induced glioma in mice, NSCs were implanted either into the tumor or at sites within the brain but distant from the tumor. When they were implanted directly into the tumor they spread through the tumor, and when they were implanted into other sites in the brain they migrated to the tumor and spread through it (Aboody et al. 2000). Even when they are delivered simply by injection into the circulation, NSCs can also target both brain tumors and tumors at other sites, including prostate cancer and malignant melanoma, without significant accumulation in normal tissues (Aboody et al. 2000).

NSCs have been genetically engineered to produce various products that could be delivered directly to the tumor (Yip et al. 2003). They can be designed to release cytolytic viruses that destroy adjacent cells, to produce antitumor proteins, or to secrete enzymes that will locally convert inactive pro-drugs into active chemotherapeutic compounds (Ostenfeld and Svendsen 2003). For example, NSCs can be made to produce the enzyme cytosine deaminase, which converts the inactive pro-drug 5-fluorocytosine into the active 5-fluorouracil. In animals treated systemically with the pro-drug, these cells are able to reduce tumor mass by 80 percent (Brown et al. 2003).

In addition to producing antitumor agents, NSCs may contribute to recovery of tissues damaged by cancer. They may differentiate directly into neurons and other damaged cell types, but they may also promote the ability of host cells to replace diseased tissue, especially if they are genetically engineered to produce appropriate neurotrophic factors. NSCs that are engineered as therapeutic agents can also be specially tagged so that they can be monitored in vivo after injection (Magnitsky et al. 2005).

Other stem cell populations with homing abilities may be useful in other kinds of cancer therapy. For example, embryonic endothelial progenitor cells preferentially localize to lung metastases and integrate in tumor blood vessels when delivered intravenously into tumor-bearing mice (Wei et al. 2004).

Cardiovascular Disease

Cardiovascular disease causes about half of the deaths in developed countries and is likely to become the leading cause of death worldwide in the near future (Mathur and Martin 2004). Stem cell transplantation may provide an inexpensive therapy for at least some of the diseases affecting the heart. Most of the cardiovascular problems begin with a myocardial infarction or heart attack, in which blockage of the coronary artery starves some of the heart muscle of oxygen and nutrients, leading to death of some of the muscle cells and the replacement of healthy muscle by scar tissue. The damaged heart is unable to pump normally, and this can lead to a syndrome of consequences called congestive heart failure. Current therapy for this disease is limited to trying to prevent the changes in ventricle structure and the congestive heart failure that follows myocardial infarction.

Stem cell therapy has been proposed as a means to replace and regenerate functional cardiac muscle, rather than just prevent further damage following a heart attack. This could be achieved either by stimulating the proliferation of the patient's cardiac stem cells or by implanting stem cells from a donor. Animal studies have already shown that injected bone marrow or fetal liver stem cells can regenerate heart muscle and improve circulation to the damaged area, suggesting that stem cell transplantation is feasible and may have beneficial effects (Amado et al. 2005; Lanza et al. 2004; Yoon et al. 2005).

Both human and animal studies have also suggested that cells originating outside the heart could be involved in its repair. In male recipients of heart transplants from female donors, biopsies have shown the presence of male cells in cardiomyocytes of the female heart, indicating that these cells originated outside the heart and from the recipient's body. The bone marrow is a likely source of such cells, raising the possibility that bone marrow transplantation could be used to supply stem cells for the diseased heart following a heart attack. The bone marrow also contains endothelial precursors that could potentially be used to induce the formation of new blood vessels in the affected area (Anversa et al. 2002; Beltrami et al. 2003; Lanza et al. 2004).

In spite of uncertainties about the experimental studies, clinical trials of bone marrow transplantation have been carried out on patients with severe heart failure (Mathur and Martin 2004). The patients' own bone marrow cells or progenitor cells from the blood were injected into specific regions of the heart or delivered via a catheter, and the patients were monitored for heart function. No adverse effects have been reported, and some improvement in cardiac function has been reported in several of the studies (Mathur and Martin 2004). It is clearly necessary to carry out large-scale, well-designed clinical trials of stem cell therapy for cardiovascular and other disorders (Mathur and Martin 2004).

Metabolic Diseases

As mentioned above, HSC therapy for metabolic diseases has had some but limited success (Malatack et al. 2003). This limit is particularly true for the central nervous system. In animal models of some of the lysosomal storage disorders, however, implantation of NSCs into the brain significantly ameliorates the detrimental effects of the disease on the brain (Eto et al. 2004; Shihabuddin et al. 2004). These data suggest that combination stem cell therapy, using HSCs for the periphery and NSCs for the brain, might be a much more effective treatment strategy for these patients. In addition, transplantation of another stem cell component of bone marrow, the mesenchymal stem cells, may be beneficial for the bone and cartilage defects found in these diseases (Koc et al. 2002).

Osteoporosis

In studies on mammalian model systems, implants containing mesenchymal stem cells have shown positive effects on tissue repair for bone and tendon (Dennis and Caplan 2003). Introduction of mesenchymal precursor cells into the circulation is also being tried as a method to counteract age-related osteoporosis or as a cure for osteogenesis imperfecta, but the cells appear in the bones and other target tissues only at a low frequency (Dennis and Caplan 2003).

AVOIDING OR OVERCOMING IMMUNE REJECTION IN STEM CELL TRANSPLANTATION

One of the major problems with transplantation of any kind is the possibility of immune rejection of the transplanted tissue. During immune rejection, the immune system of the recipient of the transplant recognizes the transplanted cells as foreign and mounts a robust response to remove them. This can result not only in the loss of the transplanted cells but also in the death of the recipient. Currently, the only way to avoid immune rejection altogether is to have the cells that are transplanted come from an identical twin of the recipient or from the recipient him-/herself (an autologous transplant). Clearly, the former happens only very infrequently. The latter can happen in the case where bone marrow is harvested from the recipient, is cleared of cancer cells—for example, in the laboratory—and then is put back into the recipient. This is also a relatively rare occurrence.

Currently, two strategies are used to prevent or reduce the extent of the destructive immune response: suppression of the immune system with drugs and careful HLA matching of the donor to the recipient. Recently, advances in ESC research have suggested a new approach: somatic cell nuclear transfer (SCNT), which is used to produce an ESC line that is derived from, and therefore theoretically immune matched to, the recipient (Lanza et al. 2004). Another approach is pretransplantation induction of immune tolerance with cells derived from the same ESC line to be used to derive the cells needed for therapy (Beyth et al. 2005; Fairchild, Cartland, et al. 2004; Fairchild, Nolan, et al. 2005). Finally, an expansion of the concept of autologous transplantation to include treatment of other tissue types provides an immune rejection–free approach.

Immunosuppression

It is anticipated that the use of stem cells from nonautologous (allogeneic) donors will require the same kind of immunosuppression that is being used with other organ transplant therapies. This is clearly true for HSCs and presumably will also be true for other adult stem cells. Immune suppression, however, may put the recipient at risk for infection, and should lifelong immunosuppression begin in early childhood, the risks are greatly magnified (Davies et al. 2005; Rianthavorn et al. 2004). There is some evidence that ESCs may not elicit the same kind of immune response that is associated with transplantation of more mature cells or tissues. Injection of ESCs into immune-competent mice failed to induce an immune response (Li et al. 2004), suggesting that any ESC line may be immunologically compatible with any recipient, obviating the need for either therapeutic cloning or a large ESC bank. These studies, however, must be replicated and expanded to include specific differentiated cell types (Li et al. 2004).

HLA Matching

HLA matching remains the single most effective method for minimizing immune rejection. With HLA matching the idea is to use donor cells with immunogenic properties that are similar to those of the recipient, minimizing the extent of immune rejection. As HLA subtypes are genetically determined, the first donors considered are the patient's siblings. Even when sibling donors are used for bone marrow transplantation, the chances of success are much higher if the donor is fully matched for HLAs. However, the chances of a sibling being completely matched are only 25 to 30 percent, so unrelated donors are often used despite high mortality rates, which are up to 40 to 50 percent in older recipients (Lewis 2002). At present, only about 70 percent of transplant patients can find an appropriate immunologically matched, unrelated donor through the National Marrow Donor Program and other similar entities that have a combined pool of six to seven million potential donors (Goldman and Horowitz 2002); the remaining 30 percent are transplanted with a less-than-ideal match and/or die (Ringden et al. 2004). Similar problems are likely to arise in other examples of allogeneic stem cell therapy.

Somatic Cell Nuclear Transfer

One solution to the potential problems of immune rejection of transplanted stem cells would be to generate stem cells genetically identical to the patient. In principle, this can be done by replacing the nucleus of a donor egg with a nucleus from a somatic (body) cell of the patient and growing up the resulting blastocyst for a new stem cell line, which could be used in stem cell therapy. This process of SCNT has been shown in animal models (Lanza et al. 2004). Since bone marrow transplants can be used successfully for treatment of some of the hematologic malignancies, and given the constraints of HLA matching, a first clinical application of ESCs produced by SCNT might well be the treatment of patients with hematologic disorders for whom a matched bone marrow donor cannot be found. Three confounders, however, threaten the apparent simplicity of this approach to the problem of immune rejection: (1) to date, only one laboratory has been successful with human nuclear transfer (Stojkovic et al. 2005), suggestive of its technical difficulty; (2) matching of the mitochondrial genome, which contributes to the minor histocompatibility complexes, is not solved with this approach (Beatty

1997; Simpson 1998), suggesting that immune rejection problems may persist after SCNT; and (3) the availability of egg donors is unlikely to satisfy the potential demand (Dickenson 2004; Magnus and Cho 2005).

Induction of Immune Tolerance

As mentioned above, even though SCNT has the potential to produce immune privileged cells that may not be recognized and therefore to avoid rejection by the host's immune system, there is still the potential of rejection due to the residual mitochondrial DNA protein products that will be produced by these cells. It is unlikely, therefore, that fully differentiated cells from ESCs, derived from in vitro fertilization (IVF) or SCNT, will fully evade immune rejection. One strategy is to use tolerogenic immune cells, derived from the ESC line from which the differentiated cells to be transplanted will be derived, to induce a state of immune tolerance in the host (Priddle et al. 2005). In this procedure, a subpopulation of HSCs, dendritic cells, would first be derived from the ESCs and transplanted into the recipient. The dendritic cells would "train" the recipient's immune system to accept other cells derived from the same ESC line (Fairchild, Cartland, et al. 2004; Fairchild, Nolan, et al. 2005). The subsequent transplant of differentiated cells would therefore not be recognized as foreign by the recipient's immune system and would not be rejected. For this approach to be successful, however, a reliable method for the derivation of dendritic cells from ESCs would have to be perfected, and the transplantation procedure for the reliable induction and validation of immune tolerance would have to be devised. One important implication of this approach is that any ESC line would be suitable for transplantation into any patient, minimizing the number of ESC lines that would otherwise be necessary for widespread use. Another implication here is that since transplantation of differentiated ESCs would have to be delayed until immune tolerance was induced, diseases or injuries that might require transplantation before that point might not be candidates for this approach.

Expansion of Autologous Transplantation

A final approach, and one that has received considerable attention, is autologous transplantation. As mentioned above, autologous transplantation is currently used when a patient's own bone marrow is removed, cleared of cancer cells, and transplanted back into the patient. In this case, bone marrow replaces bone marrow; the functions of the removed cells are identical to the functions of the transplanted cells. Recent research, however, has suggested that it may be possible to change the function of the removed cells so that, when transplanted back into the patient, they may assume new roles. Thus it may be possible to use bone marrow stem cells to treat non–bone marrow diseases such as heart and brain diseases. In this case, therefore, since the cells come from the patient who is being treated, immune rejection is not an issue. A specific subpopulation of bone marrow stem cells, mesenchymal stem cells, is already in clinical trials for the autologous therapy of heart disease and stroke.

SCIENTIFIC ISSUES ARISING IN STEM CELL THERAPY

Use of Animal Cells or Products

Feeder cells from other mammals have often been used for the culture of ESCs, and this may limit the use of the stem cells in therapy according to current FDA regulations (Klimanskaya et al. 2005). However, this regulatory hurdle can be cleared by demonstrating that the ESCs grown on nonhuman feeder cells do not carry nonhuman (or human) pathogens (viruses, bacteria). In addition, it has recently been shown that ESCs cultured in the absence of animal cells but in the presence of animal cell–derived products may show the presence of animal-specific molecules (Martin et al. 2005). Although it has been suggested that this may obviate the use of the cells for therapeutic applications, the clinical use of similarly treated cells or other implantable products has been underway for many years (FDA Xenotransplantation Action Plan). In addition, it is possible to significantly reduce the animal components simply by culture of the cells in non-animal-based systems (Martin et al. 2005).

Quantitative and Qualitative Limitations of Adult Stem Cells

Unlimited growth potential as well as multipotency distinguishes ESCs from adult stem cells. First, adult stem cells cannot yet be grown indefinitely in vitro, and this limits the number of experiments or transplantations that can be accomplished with a given cell line, although for autologous transplantation this is a minor concern. Second, because of their multipotency ESCs can be used for multiple applications, including the replacement of multiple tissues or cell types in a patient; adult stem cells do not appear to have this degree of plasticity. This is particularly important, as many diseases cause loss or abnormalities of more than one cell type. Although adult stem cells have recently been shown to have greater differentiation potential than once thought, their range of potential, at present, is much narrower than that of ESCs.

Tumor-Forming Potential of ESCs

One of the basic properties of undifferentiated ESCs is their ability to form a certain type of tumor called a teratoma. Implantation of this type of cell, therefore, carries substantial risk (Arnhold, Klein, et al. 2004). Undifferentiated ESCs are thus unlikely to be used directly in therapeutic applications. Differentiation of an ESC eliminates its capacity to form a tumor. Thus ESCs will be used to generate lines of cells that are at least partially differentiated, and these derived cell lines will be used therapeutically (Lanza et al. 2004). However, it will be important to demonstrate that no undifferentiated cells remain.

Assessing the Genetic Normality of ESCs

There is currently no way of knowing whether ESCs are genetically normal and would be safe to use in stem cell therapy (Allegrucci et al. 2004). Indeed, long-term safety studies may well take decades to complete. The technique of IVF, which provides the starting material for the derivation of ESCs, often produces genetically abnormal embryos (De Rycke et al. 2002; Niemitz and Feinberg 2004; Schieve et al. 2004). After IVF, failure to implant or tendency to miscarry is closely correlated with, and probably caused by, abnormal numbers or types of chromosomes in the cells of the embryo. Many of the chromosomally abnormal embryos are probably lost before they are even detected. However, new data suggest that IVF is associated with a high incidence of low birth weight and of genetic defects such as Beckwith-Wiedemann syndrome, Angelman syndrome, and retinoblastoma (Niemitz and Feinberg 2004; Van Steirteghem et al. 2002). In IVF clinics this problem is being addressed using preimplantation genetic diagnosis (PGD), wherein the embryos are genetically evaluated using high-sensitivity molecular techniques (amplification by polymerase chain reaction followed by DNA sequence analysis, or fluorescence in situ hybridization, or comparative genomic hybridization), and only blastocysts that show no detectable abnormalities are implanted. Application of PGD to IVF has significantly increased implantation rates, reduced spontaneous abortions, and reduced chromosomally abnormal conceptions. Similar techniques could be applied to ESCs before they are used in therapy.

ETHICAL ISSUES ARISING IN STEM CELL THERAPY

The complex ways in which transplanted stem cells may benefit the patient raise important ethical issues. For example, to anticipate the limited availability of HLA-matched siblings, at least nine couples have already preselected embryos, in an IVF setting, that would be the best tissue donors for their existing children. Embryos were screened by PGD HLA testing, and the selected embryos were implanted to create five healthy babies that could serve as stem cell donors for their siblings who suffered from leukemia or anemia (Verlinsky et al. 2004). This raises an important ethical issue, since it is the first example of the use of PGD to select embryos based on their potential benefit to others rather than on their own future health.

Other examples include clinical trials being started and stem cell treatment programs being offered without any clinical trials, involving transplantation of stem cells with very little knowledge of whether the treatment will work or about the mechanisms of any effect that does occur. At least five companies are offering stem cell therapies in countries where the regulations governing experimental procedures are less stringent than in the United States. This is bypassing the generally accepted goals of clinical trials to show, first, that the proposed treatment does not cause harm, and, second, that it is effective.

Of course, similar ethical issues have arisen in many other areas of medicine, since the precise mechanism of many new therapies, especially pharmaceutical ones, is incompletely understood. However, the issue is heightened in the case of cell-based therapies, since the mechanisms of action are likely to be much more complicated than is the case for more conventional therapies, since reversing the transplantation may not be possible, and since cell-based therapies are being promoted as a potential solution for many major injuries and devastating, progressive, and otherwise incurable diseases. In these cases the patients and their families can be desperate enough to try innovative, risky, and expensive approaches with very little proof that they will be helpful. It is difficult to deny them this one glimmer of hope. However, lessons from the gene therapy story show that the hasty application of innovative therapies can be disastrously harmful to the patient and counterproductive for the field (Grilley and Gee 2003; Rubanyi 2001; Somia and Verma 2000).

Finally, with regard to the level of optimism that has been generated over the potential of stem cell therapies to cure diseases and heal injuries, it is important that from time to time a realistic appraisal of this optimism be made. As an example, spinal cord injury (SCI) has been in the spotlight as one of the nervous system injuries that could best benefit from stem cell therapies (McDonald et al. 1999). A well-known actor, Christopher Reeve, suffered a spinal cord injury himself and became a very effective spokesperson for patients with SCI. His foundation reports that 250,000 Americans are currently spinal cord injured and that every year an additional 11,000 Americans become spinal cord injured (Christopher and Dana Reeve Foundation 2007). In a speech to supporters in Iowa on October 10, 2004, John Edwards, a Democratic senator from North Carolina and vice-presidential candidate for the 2004 election, stated, "If we can do the work that we can do in this country— the work we will do when John Kerry is president—people like Christopher Reeve are going to walk. Get up out of that wheelchair and walk again" (QuickOverview.com 2007). Thus the level of "hype" reached its maximum. Unfortunately, at that time there was not a single, published, peer-reviewed, scientific study that showed a positive effect of human embryonic stem cell therapy in any animal model of SCI, much less human SCI. Subsequently, a study published by Keirstead et al. in 2005 did show a modest effect of transplantation of cells differentiated from human embryonic stem cells in a rat model of SCI. An more important finding of that study, however, was that the effect was only seen in animals that had a recent (and moderate) injury; there was no effect seen in animals with chronic injury. The implication, therefore, is that at this time no patient with SCI is likely to benefit from this therapeutic approach; the only persons who might benefit are those that have not yet been injured and who suffer the injury in the future, after clinical trials with human ESC-derived cells have demonstrated the safety and efficacy of this therapeutic approach. This is not likely to occur for at least another five years and probably much longer than that.

REFERENCES

Aboody, K. S., A. Brown, N. G. Rainov, K. A. Bower, S. Liu, W. Yang, J. E. Small, U. Herrlinger, V. Ourednik, P. M. Black, X. O. Breakefield, and E. Y. Snyder. 2000. Neural stem cells display extensive tropism for pathology in adult brain: Evidence from intracranial gliomas. Proc. Natl. Acad. Sci. U.S.A. 97:12846–51.

Allegrucci, C., C. Denning, H. Priddle, and L. Young.
2004. Stem-cell consequences of embryo epigenetic defects. Lancet 364:206–8.

Alzheimer's Association.
2005. Fact sheet. www.alz.org/documents/national/FSAlzheimerstats .pdf. Accessed May 3, 2007.

Amado, L. C., A. P. Saliaris, K. H. Schuleri, M. St. John, J. S. Xie, S. Cattaneo, D. J. Durand, T. Fitton, J. Q. Kuang, G. Stewart, S. Lehrke, W. W. Baumgartner, B. J. Martin, A. W. Heldman, and J. M. Hare.
2005. Cardiac repair with intramyocardial injection of allogeneic mesenchymal stem cells after myocardial infarction. Proc. Natl. Acad. Sci. U.S.A. 102:11474–79.

American Diabetes Association.
2007. All about diabetes. 222.diabetes.org/about-diabetes.jsp. Accessed May 3, 2007.

American Heart Association.
2007. Heart disease and stroke statistics—2007 update. http://circ/ ahajournals.org/cgi/content/full/115/5/e69/TBL1179728. Accessed May 3, 2007.

American Parkinson Disease Association.
2003. American Parkinson Disease Association Inc. www.apdaparkinson .org/user/index.asp. Accessed May 3, 2007.

Anversa, P., A. Leri, J. Kajstura, and B. Nadal-Ginard.
2002. Myocyte growth and cardiac repair. J. Mol. Cell Cardiol. 34:91–105.

Arnhold, S., H. Klein, I. Semkova, K. Addicks, and U. Schraermeyer.
2004. Neurally selected embryonic stem cells induce tumor formation after long-term survival following engraftment into the subretinal space. Invest. Ophthalmol. Vis. Sci. 45:4251–55.

Arnhold, S., I. Semkova, C. Andressen, D. Lenartz, G. Meissner, V. Sturm, S. Kochanek, K. Addicks, and U. Schraermeyer.
2004. Iris pigment epithelial cells: A possible cell source for the future treatment of neurodegenerative diseases. Exp. Neurol. 187:410–17.

Baird, S. M.
2003. Hematopoietic stem cells in leukemia and lymphoma. In: S. Sell, ed. Stem Cells Handbook, 163–76. Totowa, NJ: Humana Press.

Beatty, P. G.
1997. National Heart, Lung, and Blood Institute (NHLBI) workshop on the importance of minor histocompatibility antigens in marrow transplantation. Sept. 16–17, 1996; Bethesda, MD. Exp. Hematol. 25:548–58.

Beltrami, A. P., L. Barlucchi, D. Torella, M. Baker, F. Limana, S. Chimenti, H. Kasahara, M. Rota, E. Musso, K. Urbanek, A. Leri, J. Kajstura, B. Nadal-Ginard, and P. Anversa.

2003. Adult cardiac stem cells are multipotent and support myocardial regeneration. Cell 114:763–76.

Berna, G., T. Leon-Quinto, R. Ensenat-Waser, E. Montanya, F. Martin, and B. Soria.
2001. Stem cells and diabetes. Biomed. Pharmacother. 55:206–12.

Beyth, S., Z. Borovsky, D. Mevorach, M. Liebergall, Z. Gazit, H. Aslan, E. Galun, and J. Rachmilewitz.
2005. Human mesenchymal stem cells alter antigen-presenting cell maturation and induce T-cell unresponsiveness. Blood 105:2214–19.

Brown, A. B., W. Yang, N. O. Schmidt, R. Carroll, K. K. Leishear, N. G. Rainov, P. M. Black, X. O. Breakefield, and K. S. Aboody.
2003. Intravascular delivery of neural stem cell lines to target intracranial and extracranial tumors of neural and non-neural origin. Hum. Gene Ther. 14:1777–85.

Brustle, O., K. N. Jones, R. D. Learish, K. Karram, K. Choudhary, O. D. Wiestler, I. D. Duncan, and R. D. McKay.
1999. Embryonic stem cell-derived glial precursors: A source of myelinating transplants. Science 285:754–56.

Brustle, O., A. C. Spiro, K. Karram, K. Choudhary, S. Okabe, and R. D. McKay.
1997. In vitro-generated neural precursors participate in mammalian brain development. Proc. Natl. Acad. Sci. U.S.A. 94:14809–14.

Burke, R. E.
2004. Ontogenic cell death in the nigrostriatal system. Cell Tissue Res. 318:63–72.

Christopher and Dana Reeve Foundation.
2007. SCI facts. www.christopherreeve.org/site/c.geIMLPOpGjF/b.1402847/k.EE60/SCI_Facts.htm. Accessed May 3, 2007.

Cottler-Fox, M. H., T. Lapidot, I. Petit, O. Kollet, J. F. DiPersio, D. Link, and S. Devine.
2003. Stem cell mobilization. Hematology (Am. Soc. Hematol. Educ. Program) 419–37.

Davies, J. H., B. A. Evans, M. E. Jenney, and J. W. Gregory.
2005. Skeletal morbidity in childhood acute lymphoblastic leukaemia. Clin. Endocrinol. (Oxf.) 63:1–9.

De Rycke, M., I. Liebaers, and A. Van Steirteghem.
2002. Epigenetic risks related to assisted reproductive technologies: Risk analysis and epigenetic inheritance. Hum. Reprod. 17:2487–94.

Dennis, J. E., and A. I. Caplan.
2003. Bone marrow mesenchymal stem cells. In: S. Sell, ed. Stem Cells Handbook, 107–18. Totowa, NJ: Humana Press.

Dickenson, D.
2004. The threatened trade in human ova. Nat. Rev. Genet. 5:167.

Drucker-Colin, R., and L. Verdugo-Diaz.
2004. Cell transplantation for Parkinson's disease: Present status. Cell Mol. Neurobiol. 24:301–16.

Ehtesham, M., P. Kabos, M. A. Gutierrez, N. H. Chung, T. S. Griffith, K. L. Black, and J. S. Yu.
2002. Induction of glioblastoma apoptosis using neural stem cell-mediated delivery of tumor necrosis factor-related apoptosis-inducing ligand. Cancer Res. 62:7170–74.

Eto, Y., J. S. Shen, X. L. Meng, and T. Ohashi.
2004. Treatment of lysosomal storage disorders: Cell therapy and gene therapy. J. Inherit. Metab. Dis. 27:411–15.

Fairchild, P. J., S. Cartland, K. F. Nolan, and H. Waldmann.
2004. Embryonic stem cells and the challenge of transplantation tolerance. Trends Immunol. 25:465–70.

Fairchild, P. J., K. F. Nolan, S. Cartland, and H. Waldmann.
2005. Embryonic stem cells: A novel source of dendritic cells for clinical applications. Int. Immunopharmacol. 5:13–21.

Furlan, R., S. Pluchino, and G. Martino.
2003. The therapeutic use of gene therapy in inflammatory demyelinating diseases of the central nervous system. Curr. Opin. Neurol. 16:385–92.

Goldman, J. M., and M. M. Horowitz.
2002. The international bone marrow transplant registry. Int. J. Hematol. 76, suppl. 1, 393–97.

Grilley, B. J., and A. P. Gee.
2003. Gene transfer: Regulatory issues and their impact on the clinical investigator and the good manufacturing production facility. Cytotherapy 5:197–207.

Grondin, R., Z. Zhang, Y. Ai, D. M. Gash, and G. A. Gerhardt.
2003. Intracranial delivery of proteins and peptides as a therapy for neurodegenerative diseases. Prog. Drug Res. 61:101–23.

Heng, B. C., T. Cao, H. K. Haider, D. Z. Wang, E. K. Sim, and S. C. Ng.
2004. An overview and synopsis of techniques for directing stem cell differentiation in vitro. Cell Tissue Res. 315:291–303.

Imitola, J., K. Raddassi, K. I. Park, F. J. Mueller, M. Nieto, Y. D. Teng, D. Frenkel, J. Li, R. L. Sidman, C. A. Walsh, E. Y. Snyder, and S. J. Khoury.
2004. Directed migration of neural stem cells to sites of CNS injury by the stromal cell-derived factor 1alpha/CXC chemokine receptor 4 pathway. Proc. Natl. Acad. Sci. U.S.A. 101:18117–22.

Keirstead, H. S., G. Nistor, G. Bernal, M. Totoiu, F. Cloutier, K. Sharp, and O. Steward.
2005. Human embryonic stem cell-derived oligodendrocyte progenitor cell transplants remyelinate and restore locomotion after spinal cord injury. J. Neurosci. 25:4694–4705.

Kelley, M. W., J. K. Turner, and T. A. Reh.

1995. Regulation of proliferation and photoreceptor differentiation in fetal human retinal cell cultures. Invest. Ophthalmol. Vis. Sci. 36: 1280–89.

Kim, D. W.

2004. Efficient induction of dopaminergic neurons from embryonic stem cells for application to Parkinson's disease. Yonsei Med. J. 45, suppl., 23–27.

Klassen, H., B. Ziaeian, I. I. Kirov, M. J. Young, and P. H. Schwartz.

2004. Isolation of retinal progenitor cells from post-mortem human tissue and comparison with autologous brain progenitors. J. Neurosci. Res. 77:334–43.

Klimanskaya, I., Y. Chung, L. Meisner, J. Johnson, M. D. West, and R. Lanza.

2005. Human embryonic stem cells derived without feeder cells. Lancet 365:1636–41.

Koc, O. N., J. Day, M. Nieder, S. L. Gerson, H. M. Lazarus, and W. Krivit.

2002. Allogeneic mesenchymal stem cell infusion for treatment of metachromatic leukodystrophy (MLD) and Hurler syndrome (MPS-IH). Bone Marrow Transplant 30:215–22.

Lanza, R., M. A. Moore, T. Wakayama, A. C. Perry, J. H. Shieh, J. Hendrikx, A. Leri, S. Chimenti, A. Monsen, D. Nurzynska, M. D. West, J. Kajstura, and P. Anversa.

2004. Regeneration of the infarcted heart with stem cells derived by nuclear transplantation. Circ. Res. 94:820–27.

Lapidot, T., and I. Petit.

2002. Current understanding of stem cell mobilization: The roles of chemokines, proteolytic enzymes, adhesion molecules, cytokines, and stromal cells. Exp. Hematol. 30: 973–81.

Lechner, A., and J. F. Habener.

2003. Stem/progenitor cells derived from adult tissues: Potential for the treatment of diabetes mellitus. Am. J. Physiol. Endocrinol. Metab. 284:E259–66.

Lewis, I. D.

2002. Clinical and experimental uses of umbilical cord blood. Intern. Med. J. 32:601–9.

Li, L., M. L. Baroja, A. Majumdar, K. Chadwick, A. Rouleau, L. Gallacher, I. Ferber, J. Lebkowski, T. Martin, J. Madrenas, and M. Bhatia, M.

2004. Human embryonic stem cells possess immune-privileged properties. Stem Cells 22:448–56.

Liu, S., Y. Qu, T. J. Stewart, M. J. Howard, S. Chakrabortty, T. F. Holekamp, and, J. W. McDonald.

2000. Embryonic stem cells differentiate into oligodendrocytes and myelinate in culture and after spinal cord transplantation. Proc. Natl. Acad. Sci. U.S.A. 97:6126–31.

Lu, P., L. L. Jones, E. Y. Snyder, and M. H. Tuszynski.
    2003. Neural stem cells constitutively secrete neurotrophic factors and pro-
    mote extensive host axonal growth after spinal cord injury. Exp. Neurol.
    181:115–29.

Magnitsky, S., D. J. Watson, R. M. Walton, S. Pickup, J. W. Bulte, J. H. Wolfe,
    and H. Poptani.
    2005. In vivo and ex vivo MRI detection of localized and disseminated neu-
    ral stem cell grafts in the mouse brain. Neuroimage 26:744–54.

Magnus, D., and M. K. Cho.
    2005. Ethics: Issues in oocyte donation for stem cell research. Science
    308:1747–48.

Malatack, J. J., D. M. Consolini, and E. Bayever.
    2003. The status of hematopoietic stem cell transplantation in lysosomal stor-
    age disease. Pediatr. Neurol. 29:391–403.

Martin, M. J., A. Muotri, F. Gage, and A. Varki.
    2005. Human embryonic stem cells express an immunogenic nonhuman sialic
    acid. Nat. Med. 11:228–32.

Mathur, A., and J. F. Martin.
    2004. Stem cells and repair of the heart. Lancet 364:183–92.

McDonald, J. W., X. Z. Liu, Y. Qu, S. Liu, S. K. Mickey, D. Turetsky, D. I. Got-
    tlieb, and, D. W. Choi.
    1999. Transplanted embryonic stem cells survive, differentiate and promote
    recovery in injured rat spinal cord. Nat. Med. 5:1410–12.

Miyamoto, M.
    2001. Current progress and perspectives in cell therapy for diabetes mellitus.
    Hum. Cell 14:293–300.

Nash, R. A., J. D. Bowen, P. A. McSweeney, S. Z. Pavletic, K. R. Maravilla, M. S.
    Park, J. Storek, K. M. Sullivan, J. Al Omaishi, J. R. Corboy, J. DiPersio, G. E.
    Georges, T. A. Gooley, L. A. Holmberg, C. F. LeMaistre, K. Ryan, H. Open-
    shaw, J. Sunderhaus, R. Storb, J. Zunt, and G. H. Kraft.
    2003. High-dose immunosuppressive therapy and autologous peripheral
    blood stem cell transplantation for severe multiple sclerosis. Blood
    102:2364–72.

National Cancer Institute.
    2006. Estimated cancer prevalence counts: Who are our cancer survivors in
    the US? http://cancercontrol.cancer.gov/ocs/prevalence. Accessed May 3,
    2007.

National Institute of Allergy and Infectious Diseases.
    2005. Progress in autoimmune diseases research. www.niaid.nih.gov/
    publications/pdf/ADCCFinal.pdf. Accessed May 3, 2007.

National Institute of Arthritis and Musculoskeletal and Skin Diseases.
    2007. Bone health and osteoporosis: A surgeon general's report. What is bone
    disease? www.surgeongeneral.gov/library/bonehealth/factsheet1.html.
    Accessed May 3, 2007.

Niemitz, E. L., and A. P. Feinberg.
2004. Epigenetics and assisted reproductive technology: A call for investigation. Am. J. Hum. Genet. 74:599–609.

Nistor, G. I., M. O. Totoiu, N. Haque, M. K. Carpenter, and H. S. Keirstead.
2005. Human embryonic stem cells differentiate into oligodendrocytes in high purity and myelinate after spinal cord transplantation. Glia 49:385–96.

Nunes, M. C., N. S. Roy, H. M. Keyoung, R. R. Goodman, G. McKhann, L. Jiang, J. Kang, M. Nedergaard, and S. A. Goldman.
2003. Identification and isolation of multipotential neural progenitor cells from the subcortical white matter of the adult human brain. Nat. Med. 9:439–47.

Ostenfeld, T., and C. N. Svendsen.
2003. Recent advances in stem cell neurobiology. Adv. Tech. Stand. Neurosurg. 28:3–89.

Pluchino, S., R. Furlan, and G. Martino.
2004. Cell-based remyelinating therapies in multiple sclerosis: Evidence from experimental studies. Curr. Opin. Neurol. 17:247–55.

Pluchino, S., A. Quattrini, E. Brambilla, A. Gritti, G. Salani, G. Dina, R. Galli, U. Del Carro, S. Amadio, A. Bergami, R. Furlan, G. Comi, A. L. Vescovi, and G. Martino.
2003. Injection of adult neurospheres induces recovery in a chronic model of multiple sclerosis. Nature 422:688–94.

Pollack, A.
2004. Many see hope in Parkinson's drug pulled from testing. New York Times, Nov. 26.

Priddle, H., D. R. Jones, P. W. Burridge, and R. Patient.
2005. Hematopoiesis from human embryonic stem cells: Overcoming the immune barrier in stem cell therapies. Stem Cells 24:815–24.

QuickOverview.com.
2007. John Edwards. www.quickoverview.com/election2008/john-edwards-overview.html. Accessed May 3, 2007.

Rianthavorn, P., R. B. Ettenger, M. Malekzadeh, J. L. Marik, and M. Struber.
2004. Noncompliance with immunosuppressive medications in pediatric and adolescent patients receiving solid-organ transplants. Transplantation 77:778–82.

Riaz, S. S., S. Theofilopoulos, E. Jauniaux, G. M. Stern, and H. F. Bradford.
2004. The differentiation potential of human foetal neuronal progenitor cells in vitro. Brain Res. Dev. Brain Res. 153:39–51.

Rice, C. M., C. A. Halfpenny, and N. J. Scolding.
2003. Stem cells for the treatment of neurological disease. Transfus. Med. 13:351–61.

Ringden, O., M. Schaffer, B. K. Le, U. Persson, D. Hauzenberger, M. R. Abedi, O. Olerup, P. Ljungman, and M. Remberger.

2004. Which donor should be chosen for hematopoietic stem cell transplantation among unrelated HLA-A, -B, and -DRB1 genomically identical volunteers? Biol. Blood Marrow Transplant. 10:128–34.

Roitberg, B., K. Urbaniak, and M. Emborg.
2004. Cell transplantation for Parkinson's disease. Neurol. Res. 26: 355–62.

Rubanyi, G. M.
2001. The future of human gene therapy. Mol. Aspects Med. 22:113–42.

Schieve, L. A., S. A. Rasmussen, G. M. Buck, D. E. Schendel, M. A. Reynolds, and V. C. Wright.
2004. Are children born after assisted reproductive technology at increased risk for adverse health outcomes? Obstet. Gynecol. 103:1154–63.

Schwartz, P. H., P. J. Bryant, T. J. Fuja, H. Su, D. K. O'Dowd, and H. Klassen.
2003. Isolation and characterization of neural progenitor cells from post-mortem human cortex. J. Neurosci. Res. 74:838–51.

Shatos, M., K. Mizumoto, H. Mizumoto, Y. Kurimoto, H. Klassen, and M. Young.
2001. Multipotent stem cells from the brain and retina of green mice. J. Regen. Med. 2:13–15.

Shihabuddin, L. S., S. Numan, M. R. Huff, J. C. Dodge, J. Clarke, S. L. Macauley, W. Yang, T. V. Taksir, G. Parsons, M. A. Passini, F. H. Gage, and G. R. Stewart.
2004. Intracerebral transplantation of adult mouse neural progenitor cells into the Niemann-Pick-A mouse leads to a marked decrease in lysosomal storage pathology. J. Neurosci. 24:10642–51.

Simpson, E.
1998. Minor transplantation antigens: Animal models for human host-versus-graft, graft-versus-host, and graft-versus-leukemia reactions. Transplantation 65:611–16.

Somia, N., and I. M. Verma.
2000. Gene therapy: Trials and tribulations. Nat. Rev. Genet. 1:91–99.

Stojkovic, M., P. Stojkovic, C. Leary, V. J. Hall, L. Armstrong, M. Herbert, M. Nesbitt, M. Lako, and A. Murdoch.
2005. Derivation of a human blastocyst after heterologous nuclear transfer to donated oocytes. Reprod. Biomed. Online 11:226–31.

Sykes, M., and B. Nikolic.
2005. Treatment of severe autoimmune disease by stem-cell transplantation. Nature 435:620–27.

Takahashi, M., T. D. Palmer, J. Takahashi, and F. H. Gage.
1998. Widespread integration and survival of adult-derived neural progenitor cells in the developing optic retina. Mol. Cell Neurosci. 12:340–48.

Van Steirteghem, A., M. Bonduelle, P. Devroey, and I. Liebaers.
2002. Follow-up of children born after ICSI. Hum. Reprod. Update 8:111–16.

Verlinsky, Y., S. Rechitsky, T. Sharapova, R. Morris, M. Taranissi, and A. Kuliev.
2004. Preimplantation HLA testing. JAMA 291:2079–85.

Vescovi, A. L., E. A. Parati, A. Gritti, P. Poulin, M. Ferrario, E. Wanke, P. Frolichsthal-Schoeller, L. Cova, M. Arcellana-Panlilio, A. Colombo, and R. Galli.
1999. Isolation and cloning of multipotential stem cells from the embryonic human CNS and establishment of transplantable human neural stem cell lines by epigenetic stimulation. Exp. Neurol. 156:71–83.

Wei, J., S. Blum, M. Unger, G. Jarmy, M. Lamparter, A. Geishauser, G. A. Vlastos, G. Chan, K. D. Fischer, D. Rattat, K. M. Debatin, A. K. Hatzopoulos, and C. Beltinger.
2004. Embryonic endothelial progenitor cells armed with a suicide gene target hypoxic lung metastases after intravenous delivery. Cancer Cell 5:477–88.

Yang, P., M. J. Seiler, R. B. Aramant, and S. R. Whittemore.
2002. In vitro isolation and expansion of human retinal progenitor cells. Exp. Neurol. 177:326–31.

Yip, S., K. S. Aboody, M. Burns, J. Imitola, J. A. Boockvar, J. Allport, K. I. Park, Y. D. Teng, M. Lachyankar, T. McIntosh, D. M. O'Rourke, S. Khoury, R. Weissleder, P. M. Black, W. Weiss, and E. Y. Snyder.
2003. Neural stem cell biology may be well suited for improving brain tumor therapies. Cancer J. 9:189–204.

Yoon, Y. S., A. Wecker, L. Heyd, J. S. Park, T. Tkebuchava, K. Kusano, A. Hanley, H. Scadova, G. Qin, D. H. Cha, K. L. Johnson, R. Aikawa, T. Asahara, and D. W. Losordo.
2005. Clonally expanded novel multipotent stem cells from human bone marrow regenerate myocardium after myocardial infarction. J. Clin. Invest. 115:326–38.

Young, M. J., J. Ray, S. J. Whiteley, H. Klassen, and F. H. Gage.
2000. Neuronal differentiation and morphological integration of hippocampal progenitor cells transplanted to the retina of immature and mature dystrophic rats. Mol. Cell Neurosci. 16:197–205.

CHAPTER 3

Ethical Issues in Human Embryonic Stem Cell Research

Philip J. Nickel

As a moral philosopher, the perspective I will take in this chapter is one of argumentation and informed judgment about two main questions: whether individuals should ever choose to conduct human embryonic stem cell research and whether the law should permit this type of research. I will also touch upon a secondary question, that of whether the government ought to pay for this type of research. I will discuss some of the main arguments at stake and explain how the ethical conflict over these questions differs from the political conflict over them. I will be guided throughout by the assumption that the unique scientific and clinical promise of human embryonic stem cell research is significant. Those who have doubts about this assumption should consult other chapters in this volume in which the issue is addressed directly.

I begin with one of the basic facts relevant to the ethical issue of stem cell research: you and I, along with everybody else we know, developed out of clumps of primordial cells, which happen to be the very same clumps that serve as the source for human embryonic stem cells in the laboratory. Let us call these "source cells" for short, since they can be used in this way. Each individual has developed into whatever she is now out of a one-celled animal, which then became a blastocyst, a multicelled human embryo. These blastocysts are partly made up of an inner mass of cells, and the body of every adult person has developed out of this inner mass. It is this very same clump from the inner part of the blastocyst that consists of source cells for human embryonic stem cell research.

These cells can be extracted and grown into a laboratory specimen of extraordinary interest to scientists.

Before discussing the significance of the fact that all humans originate from these source cells, it is useful to begin by asking some perhaps rather simple-minded questions about how any one of us knows this fact to be true in the first place. How do I know that I developed from a single cell, and then a blastocyst? In my own case, the main way I know this is that other people have told me so. I am a human—or so it is said—and scientists tell me that this is how humans develop. And I have every reason to think that scientists are telling the truth. It fits with what I know about procreative sex that between the point at which sperm meets egg and the time when the pregnant mother is carrying a fetus, there is an embryo inside her. This embryo, at one stage, becomes a blastocyst containing source cells. I take it that I was also conceived by my parents in this way and born in this way, and therefore that I too developed from a clump of source cells. These are the basic considerations that support my beliefs about the spatiotemporal contiguity of one particular clump of source cells with my present self. These beliefs come from knowledge acquired by a whole range of scientists over a considerable period of time, and this knowledge has gradually trickled down to me.

I do not *remember* being a single cell or a (part of a) blastocyst, so my belief that I developed out of a one-celled animal or a blastocyst is not based on experiential memory. One-celled organisms do not have the ability to store memories, so I am not able to recall any such memories. I do not remember when I first started remembering things; in fact, the occasion of my first memory is no doubt long forgotten. It happened before the first memories that I still remember now were impressed upon my mind. But I believe I can say with total certainty that I do not now remember, and I have never remembered, anything from the day when I was a one-celled animal, or for that matter from my blastocyst period.

Since I do not remember being a clump of source cells, it is hard for me to think of that clump of source cells as *me*. It is difficult to identify with the clump. The mere fact that the clump and I are spatiotemporally contiguous with each other is not enough to imply that *it* was *me*; it is not enough to imply, in other words, that *I* already existed so many years ago, in the form of a clump. The blastocyst, after all, did not have my mind and my awareness, or the ability to remember anything; in fact, about all it had of mine were some biological (e.g., genetic) similarities and my immediate family. Of course, it can also be said that when I am asleep and not dreaming I have no awareness of my surroundings and

I do not have experiences that can be remembered. But my mind, my memories, and my ability to remember do not go out of existence when I am asleep; they simply go into remission. The blastocyst does not have a mind in remission, with a personal history; it does not have a mind at all. From this point of view, it is highly problematic to say that you and I were once blastocysts, as if the awareness and personal history, and ability to remember, with which we now identify, already existed at that earlier time. We should instead say, less problematically, that we developed out of blastocysts.

With these thoughts in mind, we can go on to consider one of the important starting points for thinking about the ethics of human embryonic stem cell research. For many people, the central problem with stem cell research is that, had the source cells out of which you and I developed been used for stem cell research and then destroyed, then you and I would never have existed. We would never have had our lives, and we would not be doing whatever we are doing today. This fact is disturbing, since there is much that we would have lost by never existing, such as our entire lives, our children (if we have any), and so on. This, I think, is one of the basic facts that make people wary of the ethical permissibility of human embryonic stem cell research. It would seem that there are future people whose lives would never occur, were we to use human embryonic stem cells for research today. And by never having their lives occur, there is much those future people will lose. Let us call this the Loss of Future Life Problem for human embryonic stem cell research.[1]

It is important to distinguish this argument from the argument that when people use contraception, or even when they simply decide not to have procreative sex, they often thereby cause the loss of future human life by failing to cause all the possible people they could bring into existence to become actual persons with lives. The argument I am considering here does not assert that *any* action or omission that does not maximize the total amount of future life is therefore bad. Instead, the argument is that when there is a particular entity already on its way toward becoming a person, then depriving that entity of its future life, or making it lose the future life it otherwise would have had, is bad.

This way of framing the argument does not presuppose that I actually existed already—that I was already a person, namely, myself—during the blastocyst phase of my development. All that is required for the Loss of Future Life Problem is that the blastocyst is an entity with a likely *future* as a person, not that it is a person already. This is good because, as we were discussing above, the claim that a blastocyst is a person is difficult to defend: it runs into the difficulty that the blastocyst has no conscious mind, no awareness, and no personal history or ability to remember, whereas persons, of whom I am one, have minds and are identified strongly with those minds and with the associated abilities to think, remember, and have experiences.

Despite the intuitive force of the Loss of Future Life Problem, proponents of research using human embryonic stem cells can make a strong counterargument to it. To begin with, they can point out the overall consequences of doing such research: even if there is some possible future life that is lost when embryos are not implanted but are instead used for biomedical research, there is also a great deal of future life that can be *gained* because of that research—or so it is reasonable to predict. Moreover, the future life that can be gained can be gained not by merely possible people but by actual people who will already exist by the time the benefit comes to them. The potential benefits of such research to actual persons, down the road, are such as to cancel out the loss of life to merely possible persons.[2]

Most people, of course, do not regard the consequences of a particular action, in terms of pure benefit and harm, to be decisive in settling the question of whether that action is morally permissible. For example, if we could kill some actual persons in order to harvest their healthy organs, so that a greater number of other persons could live longer by having these various organs transplanted into them, the fact that there would be an overall benefit in terms of the number of years lived would hardly count in favor of the killing from a moral point of view.[3] These ends do not justify these means. So, if the Loss of Future Life Problem is a decisive moral problem for human embryonic stem cell research, then the fact that a large number of people can be saved by such research is not a persuasive refutation of that problem.

However, the particular blastocysts that are, or would be, used by researchers are not on their way to having future lives. This is because of how they are acquired. One source of blastocysts is the pool of embryos frozen during in vitro fertilization (IVF) procedures and never implanted. In this case the particular stem cells in question do not come from a creature that is currently on its way toward developing into an adult human being. Therefore, there is no loss of future life involved in the decision to use stem cells from these embryos for research. Any decision that did lead to the loss of future life has already occurred at some earlier time, through the decision of the person or persons contracting for IVF services not to implant one or more of the embryos created by the clinic. Thus the Loss of Future Life Problem does not apply to the particular human embryonic stem cells that come from this source.

Of course, the Loss of Future Life Problem can be raised as a problem for IVF practices themselves. Although the ethical question of assisted fertility is a complicated issue in its own right, it is worth discussing for a moment because of its intimate relation to the issue of embryonic stem cell research. It might be thought that when embryos are created for possible use in fertility procedures but not implanted they are being deprived of future life. In fact, however, this is not so clear. By itself, neither an egg nor a sperm can be deprived of future life because neither has the potential to develop into a whole person by itself. Hence, removing egg and sperm from persons for laboratory use does not in itself deprive any person of future life. Only removing a fertilized embryo from a woman and not reimplanting it results in the loss of future life. However, when fertilization occurs in vitro, outside the body, the fertilized egg is not being deprived of future life if it is not implanted. A fertilized embryo in vitro is not on its way toward a future life; left by itself it will inevitably die. It is only after it is implanted that that it begins on a developmental path toward personhood. Hence, not implanting an embryo fertilized in vitro does not cause it to lose future life that it otherwise would have had; rather, it simply omits to confer future life that the embryo otherwise would not have had.[4] This is quite a different thing: failing to create future life is not morally problematic in itself.

In any case, the fact is that IVF practices are currently legally permitted, and there are many spare embryos already in existence that will never be implanted. Certainly they will not lose future life by being used for research. Thus, even if we concluded that IVF practices should be stopped, we would still need to address the separate question of what to do with the extra frozen embryos that already exist. If the alternative is simply to leave them in frozen storage, then it matters quite a bit that we could instead use these embryos for the ultimate goal of saving lives.

Embryonic stem cells for research can also come from donated egg cells and from embryos that are created expressly for the purpose of generating new stem cell lines.[5] Egg cells can be fertilized in the lab, or, if we are to believe the results of an infamously fraudulent Korean study, they can be turned into quasi-embryos without fertilization, through the process of somatic cell nuclear transfer.[6] In terms of the Loss of Future Life Problem, the key question is again whether the embryo is being deprived of future life, and again the answer depends on whether the embryo is removed from a woman's reproductive system, in which case it is likely that it is being deprived of future life that it would otherwise go on to have. If fertilization takes place outside a woman's body, by contrast, then the embryo is not already on its way toward a future life, so destroying it does not deprive it of that particular future. The same goes for a quasi-embryo created outside the body.[7]

So far, we have been leaving aside the most important part of the counterargument to the Loss of Future Life Problem. The important point is that, had the stem cells that eventually developed into me been used for medical research instead, then I would have no complaint against that happening, because, after all, I would never have existed. Only existing people can be harmed through the deprivation of future life. Merely possible people cannot be harmed in this way; indeed, they cannot actually be harmed at all. This is because merely possible people do not exist. It is misleading to chalk up what I would have lost by not having developed and been born, as if the whole sequence of my subsequent life already existed, and were of value to me, before I existed. Although it matters to me now whether my future happens, this does not imply that it mattered, or should have mattered, to the blastocyst that became me, or that it should have mattered to somebody else on its behalf. This is because, at that time, what is now my future did not belong to any existing person. It only came to belong to me later, when I became a person.

I should say right away that I think this counterargument—especially the last part of it, which is conclusive in itself—is successful and that the Loss of Future Life Problem does not show that human embryonic stem cell research is morally impermissible. However, there are a couple of other approaches that the opponent of human embryonic stem cell research can take in trying to articulate her objection to the practice, and I will try to explain these now.

I will first discuss what I will call the *full moral standing* approach. The idea is that we ought not to use stem cells in biomedical research because the human embryos from which they come have full moral standing already. This can be contrasted with the approach we were just considering, which does not take a position on the moral standing of human embryos but merely asserts that human embryos are the entities out of which beings with moral standing develop. To say that some thing has full moral standing is a shorthand way of saying that the thing is worthy of moral consideration in itself, in the way that a person is, and in addition that it is not worthy merely in relation to some other thing that has moral standing. For example, if it were true that some ancient oak tree had full moral standing, then it would be the case that it ought to be respected in certain ways for its own sake. Nobody ought to sacrifice it for the sake of botanical research, or even for the sake of building a hospital—not even if it was the last tree available and there were no other building materials. But, as this example suggests, simply saying that something has moral standing does not give it moral standing. (I am in no way suggesting, for my own part, that that any oak tree actually has moral standing equivalent to that of an adult human being. My point is just that to propose that idea as a reasonable one I would need to offer an explanation of why it is the kind of thing that is worthy of moral consideration in itself.)

If it were true that human embryos had full moral standing, then one thing that I would have to do to respect them would be to refrain from tearing off pieces of them to use for my own biomedical research, even in order to save lives. We do not, after all, tear pieces off of living adult persons, or children, without their consent, to use in saving the lives of others. So it is important to ask: What is the basis of moral standing, such that we can decide whether a thing has it or not? Although this has been a subject of considerable debate, much of the debate has concerned issues that are not relevant to stem cells. For example, there has been a debate over whether what is required for moral standing is autonomy (self-governance), self-awareness ("self-consciousness," as philosophers call it), or mere sentience (consciousness) by itself. Many nonhuman animals, for example, are sentient but not self-aware or autonomous, and the debate over which of these things is the basis of moral standing carries implications for how we should treat these animals.[8] But since a blastocyst is not autonomous, self-aware, or even sentient, the nuances of that debate are irrelevant here. For this reason let us focus only on those views that do assign human blastocysts moral standing. I will consider two of these: the species view and the divine-conferral view.

I will consider the species view only briefly because it has already been considered and criticized elsewhere.[9] It holds that the basis of moral standing is membership in the human species. According to the view, any human being, even a very undeveloped, comatose, or severely cognitively impaired human being, has moral standing in virtue of species membership. This view implies that embryos, who are also members of the human species, have moral standing. Hence they are worthy of respect in the way that other humans who cannot represent their own interests are worthy of respect. In particular, because embryos cannot speak for themselves and cannot protect their own well-being, people must protect their well-being for them and must take them into account, just as they would take any other human being into account.[10]

The species view is usually criticized on the grounds that it is arbitrary. The assertion that a being has moral standing in virtue of its membership in the human species stands in need of further justification; by itself it does not render the idea of moral standing intelligible. Differences in species do not carry any obvious moral significance in themselves. This is brought out by the fact that it is perfectly imaginable that there might exist members of another species, very much like us in respect of their intelligence, way of life, and even appearance—yet these creatures would not be deemed worthy of full moral consideration by the species view because they were not members of the human species. The accidental fact that we know of no such creatures does not constitute a response to the objection because the species view implies that such creatures would not be worthy of moral consideration *if* they existed, and this seems plainly false. Since the view carries a false implication, it must be mistaken.

In addition, the species view is overinclusive. It is overinclusive because it implies that both sperm and egg, which are (haploid) members of the human species, have moral standing equivalent to that of adult humans. This seems counterintuitive. Although it would be possible to confine moral standing to diploid members of the human species, there is no justification for doing so that is not arbitrary or ad hoc.[11]

Other possible reasons might be offered to support the species view. For example, it is sometimes said that providing a guarantee of moral standing to every (diploid) member of the human species, including embryos, is conducive to mutual respect among all persons. In particular, treating embryos with respect enhances our ability to accord people dignity throughout their lives. This might be offered as a justification for treating every member of the human species, including human embryos, as having full moral standing. But what is striking about this kind of argument is that it does not support the conclusion that every member of the human species has moral standing. It merely supports the conclusion that every member of the human species ought to be *accorded* moral standing—whether or not it actually has that standing—because doing so helps to achieve better human relations all around. This is not just a quibble over wording. If a person has no other reason to regard a thing as having moral standing, besides this argument, then it will seem to her that she is being asked to participate in an elaborate pretense of respect toward an object that does not merit respect in its own right. It is especially difficult to defend this pretense when it carries high costs, such as preventing the acquisition of interesting and valuable knowledge, or preventing research that could save the lives of sick people. And in fact, since the argument depends on an unsubstantiated claim about what will lead to better human relations, it is not easy to defend.

Let us now turn to the divine-conferral view of moral standing, which holds that the reason why human embryos have moral standing is that God has conferred moral standing upon them. For example, in some Christian traditions, there is a belief that moral personhood begins at conception and that the human embryo is a member of the moral community.[12] This view is thought to be supported by Scripture and tradition. However, rather than considering the details of any particular version of the view, here I will consider what is common to its many versions.

To understand and evaluate the divine-conferral view of moral standing, it is necessary to explain what kinds of things can be said to support it. I think that religious and nonreligious persons alike would agree that the grounds for believing that God has conferred moral standing on some being come only from the following sources: from religious experience (e.g., a revelation of some kind, or the answer to a prayer) or from some text or religious authority (e.g., the Bible or a religious leader).

The important thing to note is that it does not make sense to expect that other reasonable persons will equally appreciate either religious-experiential or authority-based sources of belief. Different people have different religious experiences or no religious experiences at all; they adhere to different religious authorities or to no religious authorities at all. They are not unreasonable merely because they do not have the particular religious experience that is taken to support the claim that human embryos have moral standing or because they do not accept some particular religious authority on the matter as genuinely authoritative. Therefore, the divine-conferral view does not provide an adequate justification to these other people for the claim that we should not use human embryonic stem cells for research.[13]

Is there anything, then, that the opponent of human embryonic stem cell research can say to support the claim that human embryos have the same moral standing as adult human persons, something that ought to convince others who are initially unconvinced? I think that the answer to this question is "no." There is nothing, other than a religious or metaphysical conviction, to support this view. And one's own religious and metaphysical convictions, whatever merit one sees in them for oneself, have no rational force unless they are backed by reasonable arguments.

Moreover, simply *saying* that something has moral standing does not give it moral standing. I can say that the oak tree has moral standing, but that does not thereby make it the case that it does have moral standing. Suppose a hospital is really needed and the oak tree is the only source of lumber. Must it simply be accepted that the oak tree has moral standing and cannot be destroyed in order to build the hospital? Of course not. Because without a hospital there will be lives lost, it is terribly important to have something to say that will convince people affected by the decision that the oak tree is worthy of moral respect. Without this, one will have failed to justify why the tree cannot be destroyed for this purpose.

An alternative to the full moral standing approach is to hold that human embryonic stem cells have moral standing of a different sort from that of actual infants, children, and adult human persons. The most promising way of explaining this is to argue that the value of human embryos left over from IVF procedures is similar to the value of human body parts or recently deceased persons. We should think of human embryos, like human body parts or recently deceased persons, as having a special moral standing in virtue of their symbolic connection to a human life. This moral standing is not as strong as that attached to complete actual persons. However, it does imply obligations of care and responsibility that do not attach to ordinary property.

The best advocate of this view is Bonnie Steinbock. As a way of trying to articulate the idea of moral standing in question, Steinbock compares the standing of human embryos with the moral standing of recently deceased persons. She quotes Joel Feinberg:

> As Feinberg explains: "It would be wrong, for example, to hack up Grandfather's body after he has died a natural death, and dispose of his remains in the trash can on a cold winter's morning. That would be wrong not because it violates Grandfather's rights; he is dead and no longer has the same sort of rights as the rest of us, and we can make it part of the example that he was not offended while alive at the thought of such posthumous treatment and indeed even consented to it in advance. Somehow acts of this kind if not forbidden would strike at our respect for living human persons (without which organized society would be impossible) in the most keenly threatening way."[14]

Steinbock comments approvingly, "Just as disrespect for dead bodies can strike at our respect for living persons, so, too, I want to suggest, can inappropriate treatment or use of embryos. Embryos, as much as dead bodies, are a "potent symbol of human life," and for that reason have moral value and deserve respect, even though they lack interests, rights, and (therefore) moral [standing]."[15] Now, what is pertinent about this alternative approach to the moral value of human embryos is that we can accept it and still go on to say that human embryonic stem cell research is morally permissible. This is because of the implications of the analogy. It is entirely consistent with our idea of respect for the dead, or respect for body parts, that we may permissibly use dead bodies in research, or use body parts for research, or for organ and tissue transplantation. Likewise, it can be a way of treating a frozen human embryo with respect to employ it to help those who are alive. In fact, this act of using the embryo to save lives can have a very positive symbolic significance. Rather than letting an embryo go to waste in permanent frozen storage, or allowing an embryo that would have had no future as a human being anyway to die uselessly, it can instead come to have a new life and significance as a highly valued material that will help others to live.

Thus it does not follow from this alternative approach that human embryonic stem cell research is morally impermissible. On the contrary, this alternative approach affords us a way of investing human embryonic stem cell research with a kind of ritual significance as a way of respecting human life. Because the symbolism is plausible, it is reasonable to hold that the symbolic value of stem cell research is positive.

Still, I do not expect that resolute opponents of human embryonic stem cell research will accept the view on which using human embryos for research is a way of respecting them. They will reject the symbolism I have described and adhere instead to the view that such research involves killing human beings, or at a minimum involves something like the misuse of body parts. They will not be persuaded by the counterarguments I have given here. They will remain morally opposed to this research.

However, there is one final strategy that the opponents of stem cell research can use to try to show that we should not conduct human embryonic stem cell research. This strategy is based, not on the fact of the intrinsic immorality of human embryonic stem cell research—which has proven to be an argumentative dead end, or at least a stalemate of symbolism—but instead on the very fact that many people are offended by, or even disgusted by, such research.[16] Although others may not be rationally obligated to accept the reasons these offended people have for feeling the way they do, this does not change their feelings, and we should at a minimum accept the principle that, other things equal, we should try to avoid causing people to feel offense or disgust. In this way, the opponents of human embryonic stem cell research can appeal to their own feelings of offense as a reason for others not to conduct such research.

This line of thinking may be enhanced where government money is concerned. For if the government financially supports human embryonic stem cell research, it is, in effect, acting on behalf of all the citizens from whom it draws taxes. I think it makes sense that it compounds the offense or disgust of the person opposed to human embryonic stem cell research to know that, not only is human embryonic stem cell research going on, but furthermore it is being supported by the government *in that person's name.*

The problem, of course, is that there is a trade-off between the resentment that would be felt by those on either side of the issue if the matter were not decided in their favor. Many patients with currently incurable diseases and their advocates would resent restrictions on human embryonic stem cell research and its funding; those who maintain that such research is morally impermissible would resent the legal permissibility of such research and the effort to give it public funding. Both parties belong to the same political society, so the conflict cannot be avoided. If the issue is not to be decided through rational argument, then the problem is how to resolve the issue in some other way that the parties to the conflict can accept.

It is at this point—where straightforward moral reasoning is discontinued, and we begin to take people's moral disagreement as a given—that the issue becomes a distinctively political issue. To get past a fundamental moral disagreement, the two parties to the disagreement can adopt one of the following options within the political sphere. First, they can try to appeal to some common standard of reasoning that transcends their moral disagreement, perhaps by appealing only to beliefs and principles that they both share. Second, they can agree to disagree but accept a common procedure such as voting or judicial proceedings that they believe will resolve the issue fairly and in a way that they agree to accept, whatever the outcome, for the time being. Or third, they can fail to agree upon a common procedure for deciding the issue but continue to pursue the available means toward the outcome they desire.[17]

The issue of funding human embryonic stem cell research has been and will continue to be addressed in the second or third of these ways. If my argument in the first part of this essay is correct, there is little hope of deciding it in the first way—that is, by finding a shared set of moral premises for considering this issue and coming to a consensus, at least not in the near future. Despite this, I propose that the second way is better than the third; that is, it would be better if people could, by and large, at least agree on the legitimacy of a procedure for deciding whether to permit and to fund human embryonic stem cell research. But are there any prospects for finding such a consensual decision procedure?

Many things might count as consensual decision procedures. For example, we could decide to roll a die every ten years to determine whether human embryonic stem cell research would be funded by the National Institutes of Health for the following decade. We could decide to hold a national referendum on the issue. We could elect representatives and give them the power to decide. In my view, any of these procedures, if consented to by the vast majority of the people who have a stake in the matter, would be acceptable. (Yet I doubt that the roll of a die would, in fact, be acceptable to most people.)

However, at least one relevant alternative has certain limitations as consensual decision procedure: presidential executive order. A president is elected not merely to make a decision on a single issue but for a whole range of reasons. Although this is also true of the members of a legislature, a legislature has a formal, public procedure by which it decides individual questions. There is no counterpart in the case of an executive order.[18] This is in no way to raise a general objection to executive orders. In matters where urgent action is needed, or where some plausible and effective interpretation of the law is an administrative necessity, an executive order is perfectly acceptable. But where the executive order involves highly controversial moral issues, it is best to supplement it with legislative action.

The current rule on the permissibility and funding of human embryonic stem cell research in the United States has been determined in part by presidential executive order and in part by a congressional attachment to the yearly Department of Health and Human Services appropriations bill. The executive order is President George W. Bush's order of August 9, 2001, barring federal funding for research involving human embryonic stem cell lines created after that date.[19] The congressional amendment, called the Dickey Amendment, has been renewed by Congress each year since it was initially passed in 1996 and is meant to prohibit federal funding for scientific work that creates or destroys human embryos for research purposes. Thus the applicable federal law is a mixture of executive order and congressional act. The executive order is most charitably construed as an interpretation of the Dickey Amendment, applying it to the issue of human embryonic stem cell research.[20] The idea is that, if we confine federally funded research to existing stem cell lines, then the federal government will not be encouraging the creation or destruction of human embryos for research purposes. If the executive order is a legitimate interpretation of the Dickey Amendment, then it inherits the procedural legitimacy of that amendment.

However, the executive order is not the only reasonable interpretation of the Dickey Amendment. An alternative approach holds that it is possible, consistent with the Dickey Amendment, to allow federal funding of research using stem cell lines obtained from private, nongovernmentally funded sources. These would be derived, as discussed earlier, from embryos that are not on their way toward having future lives, such as those frozen in perpetuity after IVF treatments. The destruction of these embryos for research would then take place outside the domain of federal funding and would not involve the destruction of embryos that would have ever had future lives anyway. The research itself would take place within the federally funded domain.

Since there is more than one reasonable interpretation of the Dickey Amendment, and since the consequences of the interpretation are very significant, it is important to try to adjudicate the question through a procedure that all can agree on. However, it is not obvious that those whose views lie on different sides of this question would mostly agree in advance to the available procedures for deciding it, or perhaps even to the procedure of an open congressional debate leading to legislation. In that case, we would have already reached the third way of reaching a decision about human embryonic stem cells, where no procedure for deciding the question can be agreed upon by those who have a stake in the matter.

It is a notoriously difficult problem in political philosophy to determine what counts as agreement to a political or judicial decision procedure. Explicit acts by which a person binds himself to such a procedure are rare; on the other hand, exile and acts of genuine civil disobedience that express a definite lack of consent are also rare. A more common habitat for those who lose a struggle over political procedures is the middle zone of grudging obedience and continuing opposition. The ambiguity of this middle zone is compounded by difficulty in discerning whether people disagree with the decision procedure itself or merely with the outcome of the procedure. Because of these ambiguities, it is both important and difficult for opponents to show good faith toward one another throughout the process and even during the grudging aftermath. If possible, the procedure should be forged in a way that allows good faith to persist. That is my philosopher's second-ditch plea in this matter: if reason does not bring us to consensus over the issue of federal funding and legal regulation of human embryonic stem cell research, we might at least find a way for all parties to remain committed to the best possible shared political process as science and public opinion evolve.

NOTES

Thanks to Ron Miller and Lee Zwanziger, and to the attendees at the University of California, Irvine Conference on the Science, Ethics, and Politics of Stem Cells of May 22, 2004, for helpful comments on this paper.

1. Don Marquis advances this sort of argument as a criticism of abortion. See Marquis, "Why Abortion Is Immoral," *Journal of Philosophy* 86 (1989): 183–202.

2. As Arthur Grant has helpfully pointed out to me, the benefits of human embryonic stem cell research are not merely medical and therapeutic but also intellectual. Because of the foundational role of embryonic stem cells in human development, they are inherently fascinating from a biological point of view.

3. See Philippa Foot, "Killing and Letting Die," in *Abortion: Moral and Legal Perspectives,* ed. J. Garfield and P. Hennessey (Amherst: University of Massachusetts Press, 1984), 177–85.

4. For a detailed discussion of related issues, see F. M. Kamm, *Creation and Abortion: A Study in Moral and Legal Philosophy* (New York: Oxford University Press, 1992), and *Morality, Mortality,* vol. 2, *Rights, Duties, and Status* (New York: Oxford University Press, 1996).

5. On the issue of whether it is worse to create an embryo with the intention of destroying it than to create it for some other purpose while foreseeing that it will be destroyed, see William Fitzpatrick, "Surplus Embryos, Nonreproductive Cloning, and the Intend/Foresee Distinction," *Hastings Center Report* 33 (May–June 2003): 29–36.

6. Woo Suk Hwang et al., "Evidence of a Pluripotent Human Embryonic Stem Cell Line Derived from a Cloned Blastocyst," *Science* 303 (March 12, 2004): 1669–74.

7. Some critics raise a serious worry about the sale of embryos and egg cells on the grounds that there is undue pressure on women—financial or otherwise— to create embryos and egg cells for research and that this will contribute to an overall pattern of unfair treatment and exploitation of women. For example, it is claimed that in some of the South Korean research on somatic cell nuclear transfer, eggs were obtained from women researchers working under the lead scientist on the very study that was eventually published. It seems plausible to suggest that this practice places an unfair burden on women scientists; men obviously cannot be burdened in this way, and donating eggs requires an arduous procedure. This, I think, is a genuine reason to acquire such materials only through voluntary donation by third parties.

8. See, for example, Tom Regan, *The Case for Animal Rights* (Berkeley: University of California Press, 1983).

9. The most well-known criticism is in Peter Singer, *Animal Liberation* (New York: New York Review of Books, 1975). For a reply, see Carl Cohen, "The Case for the Use of Animals in Biomedical Research," *New England Journal of*

Medicine 315 (October 2, 1986): 865–70. See also Mary Anne Warren, *Moral Status: Obligations to Persons and Other Living Things* (New York: Oxford University Press, 2000).

10. See Robert P. George, "Stem-Cell Research: Don't Destroy Human Life," reprinted in *The Future Is Now: America Confronts the New Genetics* (New York: Rowman and Littlefield, 2002), 289–91.

11. Cf. George, "Stem-Cell Research": "Plainly gametes (sperm cells and ova) are not human beings. They are parts of other human beings. They lack the epigenetic primordia for internally directed growth and maturation as a distinct, complete, self-integrating human organism" (290). The expression *epigenetic primordia* suggests the theory of epigenesis, developed by Kaspar Friedrich Wolff in the eighteenth century, which holds (correctly) that the theory of "preformation"—the view that one of the gametes contains a tiny version or predecessor of the developing organism out of which it develops—is false and that an organism instead develops through successive differentiations of the embryo. George's point is that because neither sperm nor egg reproduces, or grows by itself into some further organism like us, neither is a human being. Two of George's main points seem questionable. First, it seems odd to say that sperm cells and eggs are parts of the people in which they reside, just as organs are. Second, it does not follow from the claim that sperm and eggs do not reproduce or grow into some further organism on their own that they are not a kind of human being in the species sense.

12. See Gilbert Meilaender, "Some Protestant Reflections," in *The Human Embryonic Stem Cell Debate: Science, Ethics, and Public Policy,* ed. Suzanne Holland et al. (Cambridge, MA: MIT Press, 2001), 141–47.

13. For a sensitive discussion of this general issue, see Kent Greenawalt, *Religious Convictions and Political Choice* (New York: Oxford University Press, 1988).

14. Bonnie Steinbock, "Respect for Human Embryos," in *Cloning and the Future of Human Embryo Research,* ed. Paul Lauritzen (New York: Oxford University Press, 2001), 21–33, quoting Joel Feinberg, *Freedom and Fulfillment* (Princeton: Princeton University Press, 1992), 53.

15. Steinbock, "Respect for Human Embryos," 29, quoting John Robertson, *Children of Choice* (Princeton: Princeton University Press, 1994), 37.

16. See Leon R. Kass, "The Wisdom of Repugnance," in Leon R. Kass and James Q. Wilson, *The Ethics of Human Cloning* (Washington, DC: American Enterprise Institute, 1998), 3–59, esp. 18–19.

17. On these issues, see Thomas Nagel, "Moral Conflict and Political Legitimacy," *Philosophy and Public Affairs* 16 (1987): 215–40; John Rawls, *Political Liberalism* (New York: Columbia University Press, 1993), and *A Theory of Justice* (Cambridge, MA: Harvard University Press, 1971); and Gerald Gaus, *Justificatory Liberalism* (New York: Oxford University Press, 1996). I thank Aaron James for discussion of this point.

18. A judicial solution shows similar drawbacks. In the case of many controversial issues, constitutional rights are often at stake, so there is a legitimate role for the courts. But this does not mean that the courts are the best place to decide morally significant political questions.

19. The president recently (in 2006) vetoed a bill that would have overturned his executive order, and Congress was unable to override this veto.

20. For discussion of this point, see President's Council on Bioethics, *Monitoring Stem Cell Research*, January 2004, ch. 2, available at www.bioethics.gov/reports/stemcell/; and George Q. Daley, "Missed Opportunities in Embryonic Stem-Cell Research," *New England Journal of Medicine* 351 (August 12, 2004): 627–28.

CHAPTER 4

Religious Perspectives on Embryonic Stem Cell Research

Mahtab Jafari, Fanny Elahi, Saba Ozyurt, and Ted Wrigley

Human embryonic stem cells derive from the inner cell mass within an early-stage embryo called a blastocyst, which forms five to six days after conception and approximates a hollow ball of roughly one hundred cells. As development continues, cells of the inner cell mass grow and differentiate, ultimately assuming the specialized characteristics of the major organ systems. Many scientists believe that these pluripotential embryonic stem cells have the potential to improve the knowledge and treatment of life-threatening diseases such as cancer, Alzheimer's disease, diabetes, spinal cord injury, multiple sclerosis, cancer, and heart diseases. However, the use of these cells for medical research presents an ethical double-edged sword in that the potential value to human life is countered by philosophical questions about the destruction of human life. Any proposed solution to this controversy is sure to conflict with the strongly held moral and religious convictions of one group or another. What has been missing in this dialogue is a dispassionate exposition covering the range of religious views on this important topic; this chapter fills that void.

The fundamental issue of the beginning of human life appears to have created an unwarranted tension between science and religion when it comes to embryonic stem cell research. Is this one-hundred-cell blastocyst a human person? Does it have a soul? Our belief systems, regardless of our educational background, influence our views with regard to embryonic stem cell research. As we consider this critical issue, it is important to note that the controversy is not over stem cell research per se but over the creation and destruction of human embryos. Even staunch opponents of human embryonic stem cell research indicate approval of other avenues of stem cell research, particularly investigations of adult stem cells. Further, many modern societies have already accepted the creation and destruction of embryos in in vitro fertilization (IVF) clinics. Some would argue that the creation and destruction of embryos for research that might lead to cures for disease is at least as justifiable as creation and destruction of embryos in IVF clinics.

Issues concerning human life have traditionally fallen in the domain of ethics or religion, with science and technology playing at best a supporting role. In the modern world, however, scientific and technological advances push even farther into these moral domains, posing greater dilemmas for those involved in policy making and implementation. Recent decades have witnessed numerous examples of the conflicts this creates. These advances further delineate natural laws and phenomena, pushing the frontiers of knowledge and modifying our fields of perception, our life experiences, and interaction with what lies outside the boundaries of our selves.

Policy discussions of human embryonic stem cell research remind us of the debates over recombinant DNA, in vitro fertilization, and pre-implantation genetic diagnosis; each debate takes us into uncharted waters. The idea that humans can interfere in a process so close to the origin of life itself is frightening to many, and for understandable reasons. It raises deeply troubling questions that have always plagued both religious and secular philosophy: What does it mean to be human? When and how does one gain moral status as a human person? When and how does one lose it? In many ways these are unproductive questions because what we mean by *human life* is itself not well defined.

In particular the "moral" aspect is difficult. Both scientific and non-scientific thought generally hold that human life begins at fertilization, yet there are profound differences between individuals and philosophical perspectives over whether that fertilized egg has the same moral status as a child or an adult. With this in mind, those involved in the debate over embryonic stem cell research view the issue through the prisms of religion, ethics, science, or some combination thereof. The question "Does the value we place on human life (its 'moral status') change as that life develops, and how?" comes to the fore because different cultures, different religions, and different philosophies give different answers.

TABLE 1. RELIGIOUS VIEWS ON THE MORAL
STATUS OF THE EMBRYO AND FETUS

Religion/Denomination	Blastocyst (to Day 6)	Embryo (to Week 8)	Fetus (to Birth)
Christianity	No explicit textual position; conventional positions given as follows:		
Roman Catholic Eastern Orthodox Fundamentalist Christian	Full moral status is obtained at conception		
Mainstream Protestant	Limited moral status (generally) given at conception		Fetus has limited moral status (with respect to mother's health)
Buddhism and Hinduism	Texts confer full moral status at conception, but karmic considerations come into play, making abortion and stem cell research possible		
Islam	Blastocysts and embryo have no moral status		Fetus has full moral status (at 120 days)
Judaism	Doctrinal positions given as follows:		
Orthodox	Blastocyst and embryo have no moral status		Fetus has limited moral status (with respect to mother's health)
Conservative	Blastocyst and embryo have no moral status		Fetus has full moral status

We show here that perceptions of the moral status of personhood, and the way those perceptions change through development, hinge on social, cultural, and religious tenets; the answers given to these questions are as varied as are religions and their denominations. It is not the goal of this chapter either to advocate for a particular set of beliefs or to reduce the issue to mere moral relativism. Instead, our purpose is to highlight critical aspects of major religious perspectives on human embryonic stem cell research (summarized in table 1).

The goal of this chapter thus is twofold. First, we discuss varying religious points of view on the beginning of human personhood. Second, we ask how these divergent views influence perceptions on and practices in biological research, including governmental regulation and funding of human embryonic stem cell research. We argue that divergent religious perspectives lie at the heart of the public controversy over stem cell research. The essence of the controversy surrounding embryonic stem cell research concerns the issue of when human personhood actually begins. As we will demonstrate, each of the major religions offers its own perspective on this issue. The lack of consensus increases the moral complexity of embryonic stem cell research.

From a purely philosophical point of view, we could present countless pages comparing the various belief systems and their views on the timing of ensoulment[1] of the fetus. Practical politics, however, is decisive, and public policies are collectively applied. What the collectivity decides regarding the start of human life—via the electoral process or other forms of decision making—leads us to confront directly these fundamental and troubling questions: Do we as a society have the obligation to protect a human life? At what age, day, or moment is the embryo considered a human person? And if we believe society is making an incorrect decision, as many do when it comes to matters of abortion or embryonic stem cell research, what is our obligation as individuals? Such complex issues are what give the debate over embryonic stem cell research a particular poignancy and urgency.

DIVERGENT RELIGIOUS VIEWS ON THE ORIGIN OF LIFE AND STEM CELL RESEARCH

In this essay we focus on the divergent views held by the world's major religions on embryonic stem cell research. Although disagreements exist among various religious traditions and within each tradition itself, their answers to these questions should provide a framework for a more productive dialogue between religious and scientific communities. Such a dialogue is needed to resolve the controversy that is hindering the advancement of this branch of science. Our analysis focuses on the major world religions and not, for the most part, on their numerous denominations. For each religion, scripture, ethical, and legal traditions are referenced to allude to the beginning of human life and the moment of ensoulment. Where present, the official consensus statement on embryonic stem cell research for that particular religion is noted.

Christianity

The Christian religions include Catholicism and the various Orthodox and Protestant churches. Christianity as a whole lacks a unified and definitive statement on when an embryo becomes a person, although fundamentalist Christians[2]—whether Protestant or Catholic—tend to be more opposed to embryonic stem cell research (Wall Street Journal Online Health-Care Poll 2005).

Christian scripture refers to God's involvement in the creation of the human being in the mother's womb, thus invoking our responsibilities toward the fetus and our consideration of its rights. This scripture does not, however, clearly address when human life begins, though the Bible does make reference to the origin of human life at the first breath and not at conception. According to the Christian tradition, ensoulment occurs when there is a physical body to ensoul (Gilbert 1996). Of course, this is a highly interpretable statement; early Christian philosophers would have had little understanding of the development of the fetus and no conception whatsoever of a blastocyst.

Christian Views on the Moral Status of Stem Cell Research   In general, Roman Catholics tend to believe that the embryo should be treated as human life from the moment of conception or fertilization and thus should be protected. The Vatican cites this as the primary reason why it is morally wrong to create or use embryos for stem cell research (John Paul II 2001). Likewise, the Eastern Orthodox perspective holds that human life and personhood begin with the zygote, whether created in situ or in vitro, because it can ultimately lead to a human life.

Protestants as a whole have no standard position regarding the status of embryos. The positions that various Protestant churches take on the status of the embryo fall across the entire spectrum. For fundamentalist sects, embryos are the weakest people among humankind and therefore should not be sacrificed to benefit others. For more moderate sects, however, the use of blastocytes for research purposes is permissible, since at this early stage of development the embryos do not possess the same moral status as that of a developed fetus or a full-born person.

Christian Views on Embryonic Stem Cell Research   For Catholics, the central moral concern with stem cell research is the source and kind of the stem cells; embryonic stem cells taken from a viable blastocyte are the most morally objectionable. The Catholic Church has less restrictive views on the use of adult stem cells, placental blood, or miscarried fetuses,[3] though it does voice concerns regarding stem cell research on embryos that have already been destroyed. According to this belief system, while the scientist may not have been involved with the destruction of the embryos and may only be using them for scientific purposes, his act is still considered morally suspect (Farley 1999).

The Eastern Orthodox tradition opposes embryonic stem cell research but accepts such research when fetuses from spontaneous miscarriages and not elective abortions are used. Orthodox Christians encourage medical research and support research on discovering alternative sources of stem cells such as adult stem cells (Demopulos 1999).

Mainstream Protestants tend to support embryonic stem cell research because of its potential therapeutic benefit but believe that embryos should not be created for the sole purpose of stem cell research, regardless of the status of the embryos. The majority of these moderate Protestant denominations balance these two divergent views by encouraging research on finding alternate sources of stem cells (Cole-Turner 1999). Fundamentalist denominations, by contrast, tend to oppose embryonic stem cell research as part of their general beliefs about the sanctity of the human procreative process. But even so, there is evidence of broad support for stem cell research among all Christian sects. A recent Wall Street Journal poll (Wall Street Journal Online Health-Care Poll 2005), for instance, found that support among religious denominations for stem cell research on human embryos ranged from 53 percent of those identifying as born-again Christian to 79 percent of those identifying as Protestant; opposition to such research was highest among born-again Christians (29 percent).

In summary, the Roman Catholic, Eastern Orthodox, and some Protestant churches believe that the zygote has obtained the full moral status of personhood and therefore should not be sacrificed for research purposes. It is worth mentioning that despite this overall consensus, a number of Catholic theologians do not support this restrictive view and support embryonic stem cell research (see Reichhardt, Cyranoski, and Schiermeier 2004).

Judaism

Under Judaism, both theological convictions and the Jewish ethical-legal tradition are brought to bear on Jewish perspectives on embryonic stem cell research. Jewish law, or halakah, is interpreted and presented by rabbis—called *poskin*—qualified to decide matters of Jewish law. Jewish perspectives on embryonic stem cell research therefore are based on these two components that are profoundly intertwined.

To understand Jewish views embryonic stem cell research, one needs to evaluate how Jewish theological convictions and the ethical-legal theory deal with such research. The salient principle of Jewish law is that life is precious and that any action that will protect life is permissible.

Jewish Views on the Status of the Embryo   Conservative and Orthodox Judaism differ on the moral status of the embryo forty days post fertilization. Conservative Judaism teaches that human life begins forty days after conception.[4] It is believed that the fetus is alive before this time but is not a person. Hence, its life need not be protected. Even after the fortieth day, the fetus does not have full rights until birth. According to Orthodox Judaism, forty days after the conception the fetus has moral rights and cannot be aborted unless this is done to protect the health of the mother. In addition, in vitro–created embryos may be used as sources of stem cells because these embryos have no moral status under Jewish law.

Jewish Views on Embryonic Stem Cell Research   Although Conservative and Orthodox Judaism differ on the moral status of the embryo forty days post fertilization, they both support embryonic stem cell research. Whereas in other religions the moral status of embryonic tissue is of paramount importance, in the Jewish tradition this factor is secondary. The main focus of Jewish bioethics is to save a life. The halakah states that to save even one life all religious laws—other than murder, adultery, and idolatry—should be abrogated. Furthermore, the Jewish tradition argues that prior to forty days' gestation, the fetus is not a human person and therefore that the destruction of such fetuses is not forbidden and is not murder. A preimplanted embryo is considered a nonensouled creature that should be respected but is not considered a human person (Feldman 1968). On the basis of these principles, the embryo may be used for research purposes that can result in life-saving efforts. Although the majority of Jewish *poskim*[5] support embryonic stem cell research, the question of whether we should create embryos for the purpose of using their stem cells, even to save a life, remains unanswered.

In summary, the protection of life is an important Jewish ideal. According to both Jewish theological convictions and ethical-legal traditions, embryos acquire human person status during their developmental process. But because there is a "cutoff date" set at forty days, it is permissible to use embryonic tissues, from aborted fetuses and from preimplanted embryos, for therapeutic research purposes. Thus the majority of Jewish denominations support stem cell research because it could potentially cure diseases and save lives (Dorff 1999; Zoloth 2001).

Islam

There are three major sources in the Islamic legal system: the Quran, Sharia, and *ijtihad*. The Quran is considered to be the divine revelation and thus is the prime authority in Islamic law. Its jurisdiction is analogous to that of the Supreme Court in the sense that it has precedence over any other interpretation. However, the Quran is neither an encyclopedia nor a blueprint that provides specific information about how God views each moral problem, issue, or situation (Maguire 2001). For that reason, Islamic scholars turn to other sources in the Islamic legal system when making rulings on issues that are not revealed in the Quran. The second source of Islamic jurisprudence, Sharia, comprises the law system inspired by the Quran; the Sunna and Hadith (acts and sayings of the Prophet); older Arabic legal systems (such as the Bedouin law); and work of Muslim scholars over the first two centuries of Islam (Kjeilen 1996). The third source is *ijtihad*, the research and deliberation of qualified Islamic scholars on issues that are not addressed in the Quran (Islamic Institute 2001). The rulings that come out of *ijtihad* should be consistent with Quranic principles and take into account benefits to humanity. It is important to remember that there is no papal figure or ruling class in Islam that can impose its views on all Muslims or intervene in the practices of governments in Muslim countries. (The only possible exception may be a radical Islamist government that strictly follows Sharia law.) Therefore, the beliefs and practices of Muslims on issues of reproduction and embryonic stem cell research are more diverse than what is reflected in this essay.

   To understand the Islamic perspective on stem cell research, one needs to look at how the Islamic legal system deals with the status of the embryo. Despite the regional diversity noted above, there is relatively little debate among Islamic scholars on the status of the embryo. Chapter 23, verses 12–14 of the Quran read: "We created *[khalaqna]* man of an extraction of clay, then we sent him, a drop in a safe lodging, then we created of the drop a clot, then we created of the clot a tissue, then we created of the tissue bones, then we covered the bones in flesh; thereafter we produced it as another creature. So blessed be God, the best of creators *[klaliqin]*" (Sachedina n.d.).

This passage has been interpreted as to suggest that the embryo cannot be perceived as a human being until it has developed further biologically (Weckerly 2002). The Quran does not say exactly when the soul enters the body. However, a Hadith says that "the soul is breathed into the body" when the fetus is 120 days old in the womb (Syed 1988). Since the embryonic stage runs from conception to the end of the eighth week (fifty-six days), according to Islam the embryo does not have a soul and thus is not a human being, whether grown in a petri dish (in vitro fertilization) or inside the uterus of a mother (natural environment) (Syed 1988).

Despite the understanding shared by the majority of Islamic scholars on the status of the embryo and ensoulment of the fetus, some scholars have taken a different stance on the issue. Imam Al Ghazali in his *Ihy' Ulum al Din* described human existence as occurring in stages, the first stage beginning with the settling of the semen in the womb, the disturbance of which would be a crime (Ahmad 2003). Even if one were to adopt this relatively conservative interpretation of when life begins, there is a difference between fertilization in a laboratory dish and fertilization in the womb of a mother (Siddiqi 2001).

Islamic Views on Embryonic Stem Cell Research   Islamic jurisdiction has long supported the treatment of infertility. Infertile couples seeking treatment for their problem are not seen as going against Islamic laws (Ahmad 2003). In that sense, in vitro fertilization is seen as a legitimate technique to treat infertility and is allowed as long as the fertilization is done with the sperm of the lawful husband during the couple's married life (Siddiqi 2001). The debate among scholars arises, not regarding whether IVF is in accordance with religious laws, but rather regarding how to treat the remaining embryos. Assisted reproductive technology often results in excess embryos that are not transferred into the uterus of the mother. There are three basic ways of dealing with this issue. First, the couple can spare those embryos to donate to other infertile couples. But this option would be impermissible according to the Islamic law because surrogacy (implantation of an embryo into the womb of another woman who is not legally married to the man from whom the sperm was taken) is held to be illegitimate. Similarly, transferring an excess embryo into the uterus of another woman would also be illegitimate, since it would involve a third party to whom the husband was not legally married (Ahmad 2003). This leaves two options for a Muslim couple who have undergone fertility treatment and are left with excess embryos: to discard the remaining embryos or to donate the embryos for research purposes. The Islamic Institute has convened a panel of experts to develop an Islamic perspective on stem cell research. At the end of the deliberations the Islamic Institute issued a statement saying, "It is a societal obligation to donate those extra embryos for research instead of discarding them" (Weckerly 2002).

The survey data available on the attitudes of ordinary Muslims toward stem cell research indicate that there is general support by Muslim Americans for embryonic stem cell research. The Islamic Institute's poll among 629 Muslim Americans revealed that 62 percent of survey participants supported embryonic stem cell research. Seventy-three percent of the respondents stated that they supported using embryos that had been donated after in vitro fertilization procedures, and 49 percent said it was acceptable to produce embryos specifically for stem cell research purposes. Also, 69 percent of the respondents said that the federal government should fund embryonic stem cell research (Islamic Institute 2001).

Unlike the Catholic Church and many American evangelical Christians, who tend to favor strong restrictions on embryonic stem cell research, most Islamic scholars have ruled that embryos terminated for medical reasons within 120 days of conception can indeed be used for research concerning life-saving treatments.

In summary, the Quran and other sources of Islamic law can be used to support embryonic stem cell research.

Buddhism and Hinduism

It is often difficult to find definitive statements of Buddhist or Hindu religious thought. The Buddhist and Hindu perspectives on embryonic stem cell research are no exception. Aside from certain central texts—the words of the Buddha passed down in the Pali canon and the teachings of Krishna recorded in the Bhagavad Gita, the Upanishads, and the Brahma Sutras—the faiths are split along major and minor philosophical divides, with no central authority to dictate opinion. However, the more frequently cited works that deal with the moral and philosophical issues surrounding embryos and medicine (Keown 1995, 2000; Lafleur 1992; Crawford 2003; Coward, Lipner, and Young 1988) all note that the primary texts of both religions clearly place the beginning of life at the time of conception. Indeed, Keown (1995) makes the comparison explicit. In Buddhism, conception is held to occur after intercourse if "an intermediate being" is present to descend into the womb, while the Hindu texts use the more specific term *jiva*, or individual soul, which descends into the union of semen and menstrual blood. The biological union, the fertility and virility of the respective partners, and the spiritual presence of the unborn are all equally necessary for conception to occur and gestation to begin.

Unfortunately, there is little available in the literature that directly addresses stem cell research. The argument above is generally offered in discussions about the ethics of abortion to show that Buddhism and Hinduism alike tend to be strongly prolife. Yet unlike the more familiar discussions that occur in Christian contexts in the United States, discussions among Buddhists and Hindus do not simply or even primarily concern the life and the rights of the fetus. Instead, debates about embryos and medicine tend to focus on two articles of faith that both religions share: the doctrine of karma and the doctrine of ahimsa.

Karma is a casual word in English, sometimes defined (inappropriately) as fate, but in Eastern philosophy it has a more specific meaning. Its literal translation would be "doing" or "action"; it is used to indicate what might best be described as a moral or spiritual equivalent of Newton's laws. Thus Pantajali's Yoga Sutras (Coward, Lipner, and Young 1988) claim that all our thoughts and actions leave memory traces that can then be triggered and reinforced, leading us to repeat the same behaviors, while Buddha's discourses frequently remind us that each of our acts will produce a reaction in the world around us. A skillful practitioner of either faith will take care of the momentum inherent in his thoughts and actions, the way an aeronautical engineer would account for all the forces and inertias involved in making a plane fly. One way of achieving this skillful practice lies in the principle of *ahimsa*—a term generally translated as "nonviolence" or "non-injury." Ahimsa is a compassionate proscription against hurting any living being, similar to the "do no harm" clause of the Hippocratic Oath, except abstracted as a general moral principle. Unlike the Hippocratic Oath, however, ahimsa is not concerned solely with the harm done to others but also with the karmic burden—the complex reactive chain of consequences—that is created by any such action.

Given that the embryo is considered a living being from the moment of conception, ahimsa requires that no harm be done to it. However, the same concern is given to the mother and other concerned parties, making for a complex moral calculus. Most Buddhist and Hindu sects, for instance, believe in reincarnation—harm is done to the embryo only because it is forced to reincarnate into another existence immediately and denied the opportunity to relieve or add to its own karmic burden in this lifetime. Some sects go further, claiming that the intermediate being or *jiva* cannot fully embody until all the outer coverings of humanity are present, with a developed physical form and the beginnings of mental activity, a point sometimes calculated as late as the end of the second trimester. For them, the karmic consequences of acts done to an embryo are minimal and easily balanced by other factors. The main concern, then, is whether the parents and the doctors involved believe they are creating positive karma, or at least preventing the creation of deeper harm.

These concerns become matters of lengthy debate in cases—such as abortion, around which most of the literature revolves—where a fetus is merely destroyed. For the purposes of stem cell research and similar medical practices, however, ahimsa becomes a much less contentious point. Crawford (2003), speaking from the Hindu perspective, argues convincingly that in vitro fertilization and embryo transfer are in no way negative karmic acts. Since the bulk of embryonic stem cells used in research are surplus cells donated by the parents, and since the doctors using the cells are researching medical procedures, the positive acts of having tried to bring a child to life and attempting to ease the suffering of others weigh heavily in the karmic balance. These issues have barely entered into Hindu and Buddhist moral debates, but it seems clear that the discussion in both faiths will not center on the question of whether the fetus is a living person; most Buddhists and Hindus would take that assumption as fact. Instead, the arguments will focus on the needs and intentions of the donors and the scientists involved and the potential recipients of the cures that are developed, to ensure that the most compassionate course for all is followed.

CONCLUSION

In discussing religious views toward the beginning of life, and by extension toward the religion's views of embryonic stem cell research, it is important to recall how deeply personal a religious belief is and how varied the world's religious sects are. With this caveat in mind, however, some general statements can be made about embryonic stem cell research. According to the Catholic faith and some Protestant religions, the zygote is a human person that should not be destroyed in the course of research. This stance explains their broad opposition to embryonic stem cell research. Muslims, Jews, and the majority of Protestants, by contrast, argue that the zygote is neither a human nor an ensouled person and therefore can be used in embryonic stem cell research without moral qualms, though undoubtedly this position is tempered by other moral and aesthetic issues. Finally, Buddhists and Hindus generally take the zygote to be a person, but they concern themselves more with the ramifications to spiritual life than with those to physical life. Embryonic stem cell research is acceptable so long as it satisfies ahimsa.

Every religion has an esoteric and an exoteric dimension. The exoteric—or outer—dimensions of religions vary from one religion to the next and from one region to the next because of the influence of a multitude of social, cultural, political, philosophical, and even geological considerations. Time and history will bring faiths with the same root to produce different flowers, as the saying goes, and the result is the wide variety in rituals, practices, and beliefs evident in the world today. The esoteric or inner dimensions of all religions, however, are unified in their belief that there is more at issue here than mere physical embodiment and that—whatever else might be said—the proper attitude toward living beings is one of reverence and compassion.

Medical science has ventured into areas that traditionally have been the sole province of religious belief. On an exoteric level, this is bound to have all the effects of a tiger appearing in the midst of a dinner party. What have been amiable, millennia-long discussions about the nature of life and birth are now confronted by the cold, analytical, authoritative glare of the doctor looking down through his microscope. This is bound to unsettle some, drive others into loud protestations of their own beliefs, and sow confusion in everyone as people try to reevaluate their deeply held beliefs in light of a science that few will ever fully understand. What is lost in this cacophony, though, is that the mainstream medical profession shares the reverence and compassion for life that marks religious faith. On the esoteric level there is only one goal, and though it may express itself differently in medicine and faith, there is that much common ground with which to work.

From the outset, theological issues surrounding stem cells have been as far-reaching as the technology itself. Theological implications have already helped frame the national debate and have influenced how research is conducted and funded. Nor will these theological issues go away; they are an established and settled element of the discourse. However, it must be remembered that the science of embryonic stem cells is not and never was intended to disturb deeply held religious beliefs. Debate arises only as all sides try to discover the most ethical and compassionate approach to truly worthy human aims.

NOTES

1. *Ensoulment* is a religious term referring to the inception of a soul within a human being or other creature. In general we prefer to speak of the moment when the fetus takes on moral status as a human individual, which we see as a more general category; the notion of a soul has varying meanings in different faiths, so *ensoulment* is not an unambiguous term. However, it is the conventional term, and we will continue to use it for brevity.

2. *Fundamentalism,* here and elsewhere, refers to a strict or literal reading of their central text(s), as opposed to those that allow for various interpretations and modernized readings.

3. Use of fetal tissue from miscarriages does raise a new direction of debate concerning abortion, which is wholly unacceptable in the Catholic tradition.

4. The significance of forty days is unclear. Some have suggested that it reflects the fetal "quickening," or point at which the fetus first begins to move—usually commencing after the seventh week. It is worth noting, however, that the number forty carried special meaning to the authors of the Bible: the great flood lasted for forty days, the Hebrew tribes wandered in the desert for forty years, and Moses spent forty days on the mountain; even Jesus spent forty days wandering in the wilderness.

5. A *posek* (plural, *poskim*) is a rabbi whose decisions are considered authoritative and effectively incontestable; in the practice of Jewish law, *poskim* are the ones consulted to resolve otherwise intractable debates.

REFERENCES

Ahmad, Norhayati Haji.
    2003. "Assisted Reproduction—Islamic Views on the Science of Procreation." *Eubios: Journal of Asian and International Bioethics* 13:59–60.
Cole-Turner, Ronald.
    1999. Testimony before the National Bioethics Advisory Commission, May 7. In *Ethical Issues in Human Stem Cell Research,* vol. 3, *Religious Perspectives.* Rockville, MD: National Bioethics Advisory Commission, June 2000, available at www.georgetown.edu/research/nrcbl/nbac.stemcell3 .pdf. Accessed Jan. 12, 2007.
Coward, Harold G., Julius J. Lipner, and Katherine K. Young.
    1988. *Hindu Ethics: Purity, Abortion, and Euthanasia.* Albany: SUNY Press.
Crawford, S. Cromwell.
    2003. *Hindu Bioethics for the Twenty-First Century.* Albany: SUNY Press.

Demopulos, D.

1999. "An Eastern Orthodox View of Embryonic Stem Cell Research." Testimony before the National Bioethics Advisory Commission, May 7. In *Ethical Issues in Human Stem Cell Research*, vol. 3, *Religious Perspectives*. Rockville, MD: National Bioethics Advisory Commission, June 2000, available at www.georgetown.edu/research/nrcbl/nbac.stemcell3.pdf. Accessed Jan. 12, 2007.

Dorff, E. N.

1999. "Stem Cell Research." Testimony before the National Bioethics Advisory Commission, May 7. In *Ethical Issues in Human Stem Cell Research*, vol. 3, *Religious Perspectives*. Rockville, MD: National Bioethics Advisory Commission, June 2000, available at www.georgetown.edu/research/nrcbl/nbac.stemcell3.pdf. Accessed Jan. 12, 2007.

Farley, M.

1999. "Roman Catholic Views on Research Involving Human Embryonic Stem Cells." Testimony before the National Bioethics Advisory Commission, May 7. In *Ethical Issues in Human Stem Cell Research*, vol. 3, *Religious Perspectives*. Rockville, MD: National Bioethics Advisory Commission, June 2000, available at www.georgetown.edu/research/nrcbl/nbac.stemcell3.pdf. Accessed Jan. 12, 2007.

Feldman, D.

1968. *Birth Control and Jewish Law*. New York: New York University Press.

Gilbert, Meilaender.

1996. *Bioethics: A Primer for Christians*. Carlisle: Paternoster.

Islamic Institute.

2001. "A Muslim Perspective on Embryonic Stem Cell Research." *Issues* 2, no. 3. www.islamicinstitute.org/i3-stemcell.pdf.

John Paul II.

2001. "To the President of the United States of America, H. E. George Walker Bush." July 23. www.vatican.va/holy_father/john_paul_ii/speech/2001/july/index.htm. Accessed January 6, 2007.

Keown, Damien.

1995. *Buddhism and Bioethics*. New York: St. Martin's Press.

Keown, Damien, ed.

2000. *Contemporary Buddhist Ethics*. London: Curzon.

Kjeilen, Tore.

1996. "Sharia." In *Encyclopedia of the Orient*, LexicOrient Web site. http://i-cias.com/e.o/sharia.htm. Accessed January 6, 2007.

Lafleur, William R.

1992. *Liquid Life: Abortion and Buddhism in Japan*. Princeton: Princeton University Press.

Maguire, Daniel C.

2001. "Contraception and Abortion in Islam" (excerpt from ch. 9 of his book *Sacred Choices*). The Religious Consultation on Population, Reproductive

Health and Ethics, www.religiousconsultation.org/islam_contraception_
abortion_in_SacredChoices.htm. Accessed January 6, 2007.

Reichhardt, T., D. Cyranoski, and Q. Schiermeier.
    2004. "Religion and Science: Studies of Faith." December 8. News@
    Nature.com. www.nature.com/news/2004/041206/full/432666a.html.
    Accessed January 6, 2007.

Sachedina, Abdulaziz. n.d. "Islamic Perspectives on Cloning." www.people.vir-
    ginia.edu/~aas/issues/cloning.htm. Accessed January 6, 2007.

Siddiqi, Muzammil.
    2001. "An Islamic Perspective on Stem Cell Research." www.pakistanlink
    .com/religion.html. Accessed 2004.

Syed, Ibrahim B.
    1988. "An Islamic Perspective on Stem Cell Research in Brief." www.irfi.org/
    articles/articles_1_50/an_islamic_perspective_on_stem_c.htm. Accessed
    January 6, 2007.

Wall Street Journal Online Health-Care Poll.
    2005. "Wall Street Journal Online/Harris Interactive Health-Care Poll."
    June 7. www.harrisinteractive.com/news/newsletters/wsjhealthnews/
    WSJOnline_HI_Health-CarePoll2005vol4_iss11.pdf.

Weckerly, Michele.
    2002. "The Islamic View on Stem Cell Research." September 30. www
    .camlaw.rutgers.edu/publications/law-religion/new_devs/RJLR_ND_56
    .pdf. Accessed January 6, 2007.

Zoloth, L.
    2001. "The Ethics of the Eight Day: Jewish Bioethics and Research on
    Human Embryonic Stem Cells." In The Human Embryonic Stem Cell
    Debate: Science, Ethics, and Public Policy, ed. Suzanne Holland, Karen
    Lebacqz, and Laurie Zoloth. Cambridge, MA: MIT Press.

CHAPTER 5

Political Issues in the Stem Cell Debate: The View from California

Lawrence S. B. Goldstein

This volume is about the intersection of ethics, politics, and policy with science. It is not focused on ethical issues surrounding the use of cells derived from early human embryos (hES cells) in research and treatment of disease. Thus I will not discuss the various issues in the ethical debate other than somewhat peripherally. I will, however, state that I am somewhat biased on these issues, as I do have a personal opinion about the ethical issues and how they affect the more controversial aspects of this work. In this regard, I am a basic biomedical scientist who is interested in understanding and treating human disease. I have, to the best of my ability, thought through the ethics of these issues. At the end of that process, I have concluded that my commitment in trying to help people who have the terrible diseases I want to treat outweighs our social and ethical responsibility to an early human embryo. Part of my view comes from the obvious fact that the embryos in question are simple clusters or balls of cells that have been generated in a dish in the lab, have never been in a woman's body, and are thus not pregnancies or fetuses. Such embryos (actually blastocysts as I will define them below) are at a developmental stage before any organs such as the heart or nervous system have yet formed and are capable of being frozen and thawed—not typical attributes of "people" as most of us define them. I do not believe that my opinion on this issue should earn me a comparison with the Nazis, as some have argued. I just disagree with other people who have different views.

WHY IS RESEARCH WITH HUMAN EMBRYONIC STEM CELLS IMPORTANT TO SCIENCE AND MEDICINE?

I will start with a pragmatic approach to illustrating the issues. As a scientist in California, what do I see as the potential benefits and value of human embryonic stem (hES) cell research to scientific and medical research for the state of California?

The benefit that is most focused upon is the generation of much-needed cells for transplants, what you might think of as cell-replacement therapy. But the uses of hES cells go far beyond that. Indeed, the most important uses of these cells may be for making the jump from studying human disease in animal models, which, after all, are just *animal* models, to actually working with human materials to understand these diseases. Humorously we sometimes say, "We have cured cancer in the mouse thousands of times." But that has not translated to curing cancer in humans. That is because the details of human physiology are sufficiently different that the translation from animals to humans is difficult. Research with hES cells is one approach from which many scientists see potential benefits for facilitating that translation. These stem cells may also help to develop a sophisticated understanding of genetically complex diseases or genetically complex responses to drugs. All of us have different susceptibilities to diseases and different sensitivities to drugs, gene transfer, and gene therapy. Research with hES cells may help us solve these issues.

Further, these cells may help with the rapidly increasing problem of obtaining sufficient clinical trial populations in the field of drug development. There may not be enough people to test all of the new drugs we would like to test in the coming years, so we need some other way to prioritize drugs for testing in human patients.

In my own laboratory, we have conducted research work using animal models of Lou Gehrig's disease. This research has led us to think that hES cells will be useful in the development of treatments for the same disease in humans. In fact, I hope we will be able to begin this transition in the next few years. In an additional and important approach, we are setting up research with hES cells to begin testing hypotheses about the mechanisms that cause Alzheimer's disease, for which the animal models have provided far less insight than is needed. This work will let us go beyond the limitations of animal models in studying disease physiology. For these reasons and more, I believe, we need to work in this area.

POLICY ISSUES

These considerations lead us to policy issues. One important issue is that as a scientist, I need to do research. My research is supported by both private money and public money. Where will I secure funds to support hES research? This question brings us to the argument about whether public funds should be allowed for research that some, but not all, people find objectionable. The government does many things that some of us find objectionable and that some of us agree with. The way we settle the disagreement is not by saying that the government may not do things that some people find objectionable, for then the government would do next to nothing. While some people would find this to be a good thing, I believe it is the wrong way to proceed.

With respect to research, what is the value of public funding?

The first and perhaps the most important feature of value is in the area of policy. In this country, government involvement in the financing of research activity effectively opens that research activity to public scrutiny. When research is carried out with private money, it can remain secret, particularly when it is funded and carried out in a biotechnology or pharmaceutical company. In this case, the research work often doesn't see the light of day, and society at large can have little or no idea what is going on. One way that our system has of ensuring transparency is that when the government is involved in financing the research, particularly in public institutions, there is an enormous amount of "sunshine," or oversight, including ethical review of that activity. Recombinant DNA is an example of an area in which government (i.e., public) involvement in funding since the 1970s has ensured substantial public information and input about the research.

A second area of value is the relatively unique ability of the public academic and research sector to effectively carry out critical fundamental or basic research. While an enormous amount of money in the private sector is dedicated to research and development, it tends to focus far more heavily, and increasingly, on development rather than on the initial basic research necessary for long-term discovery and development. Furthermore, the research pursued in the private sector tends to occur far later in the pipeline. Early-stage research that can lead to an understanding of basic principles, which then will lead to the understanding or treatment of disease, is largely done with public money. In this country, the mechanism for driving such fundamental discoveries is the National Institutes of Health (NIH), which funds the basic science engine that ultimately drives the biotechnology and pharmaceutical industries. We can agree or disagree as to who is capturing the most benefit from this arrangement or even whether it is the best way for our society to do things, but that is a different discussion. The facts at the moment are that the private sector generally does not invest in early- or even sometimes advanced-stage research. Even if a project is halfway through the pipeline to a drug, device, or other product, it can be difficult to get money to do something from the venture community unless the likely profit return is expected to be large. Many worthwhile studies will not be funded in the private sector if, for example, the likely patient population is not large enough, or if the intellectual property climate is too complex.

A third point is also a policy issue. If you want the best scientists involved in the development of a field of science, you're probably going to need public funding. There just isn't enough private or philanthropic support to compare to what the government puts into research at earlier stages. Most of our best scientists are in public institutions such as the University of California, Irvine. Even an institution such as Stanford, which is a private institution, is largely a public entity because of its ties to the government through various sorts of funding.

SCIENCE ISSUES

A lot of basic research is needed to make the transition from benchwork to the development of a clinically useful therapy. There are many good examples in the pharmaceutical world of drug development programs that started prematurely, without an adequate understanding of the basic human biology required to undertake them. As a result, in some cases, hundreds of millions, or perhaps billions, of dollars were spent on clinical trials for drugs that failed. In my opinion, had there been an adequate biological and scientific understanding of the principles underlying how particular drugs were to be used, we could have avoided much of the expenditure, wasted human resources, and participation by subjects in unnecessary clinical trials.

A second scientific issue, previously mentioned, is that human and animal cells don't always behave the same way. The principles by which animal cells operate are similar, and sometimes nearly identical, to the principles by which human cells operate. Imagine, however, that you were a car mechanic and that you spent your entire life fixing Volkswagens. If someone were to drive in with a Cadillac for repair, you simply wouldn't have the necessary tools. The tools you would have for Volkswagens wouldn't necessarily work on a Cadillac and, certainly, the parts from a Volkswagen wouldn't fit in the same place in the Cadillac. There is an analogous situation with animal cells and human cells. In fact, if I wanted to cure diabetes in the mouse, I would work on the mouse. But my goal is not to cure diabetes in the mouse but to cure it in the human. At some point, you have to work with human materials to do that. In my view, the earlier you work on human tissue the better because that allows you to combine the research and the development phases of the scientific research that you're conducting.

These are some of the reasons why, from a policy and scientific standpoint, and from my perspective as a practicing scientist, you need to have public funding involved with an endeavor like this.

SOCIETAL ISSUES

What are some of the social issues in this debate? We have already touched on some of them, but I think that the most important issue is the controversial moral status of the early human embryo, in particular the human blastocyst. The blastocyst is a hollow ball of cells that develops a few days after fertilization and has no organs such as a heart or a nervous system. If implanted into a woman's uterus, it can initiate a pregnancy and develop into a fetus. Some people view the destruction of the human blastocyst to obtain cells as murder, and there is no way that we are going to get beyond that in some people's belief systems. There are those among us who believe this, and we may not ever change the minds of those people. I and many other people of good conscience disagree with this opinion. I thus will remind you that we live in a pluralistic society. We are diverse—religiously and ethically—and moral and ethical people of good conscience can disagree. In California, which is a democracy, and the United States, which is a democracy, we vote and then we live with the consequences. I see no other way of deciding this issue. I am not morally callous; however, I will ask whether most Americans think that a hollow ball of two hundred human cells that has no heart, blood, brain, or other tissues, and that is growing in a dish or frozen in a freezer in a laboratory, is a person. I do not think that most Americans believe that these frozen balls of cells are people.

What you might think of as public antipathy toward cloning also plagues this debate. People don't like cloning—at least that's what they tell us. Cloning just means copying things. For example, we clone or copy software. We also clone human DNA—that's what gave us human insulin, human Epo [Erythropoetin], and other wonderful therapeutic agents. We also routinely clone human cells to study cancer treatments. Part of the problem in my view is essentially the problem of language. One person's baby is another person's blastocyst in this debate. When I've debated with people who believe that a blastocyst is a person, they have sometimes referred to it as a baby. I just don't agree with this point of view, so I refer to it as a blastocyst, which is precise and has no legal or scientific ambiguity. Regardless, the language has a large impact on how this issue is perceived by people. It has had an enormous impact in California, where, I will argue, the population of the state has become reasonably educated because there has been movement on these issues.

LEGAL ISSUES

I turn now to the legal issues and legal precedents in California and, indeed, in the rest of the United States.

First, as a matter of legal precedent, although a great number of people disagree with the law, abortion is legal in this country. Unless that situation changes, it is the law, and we live by the law. Second, the destruction of human blastocysts or embryos during and after in vitro fertilization and their indefinite storage in freezers, which I will argue is equivalent to destruction, are completely legal. They occur on a daily basis and can be pursued as long as public funds are not involved. The withholding of public funds, in this case, is not having an impact on whether human blastocysts are created, destroyed, or stored in freezers. The question, given that this is happening, is whether it is appropriate for the public to sanction this activity by providing public funds.

You will recall that President Bush, when he was a candidate, said decisively that he would not allow public funding for human embryonic stem cell research. After election to office, and after consulting experts in the relevant scientific and ethical fields, President Bush conceived a plan that attempted to balance the conflicting views. The balance was imperfect in the eyes of most. Both proponents and opponents of the research were dissatisfied with the approach taken. Under President Bush's plan, federal funds can be used for research with human embryonic stem cells, and he announced that there also would be robust funding for both embryonic and adult stem cell research. While there is, and has been for years, substantial funding for adult stem cell research, funding for work with human embryonic stem cells has materialized somewhat slowly. A problem in the eyes of many is that President Bush's plan included a number of restrictions on the use of stem cells derived from human blastocysts. Most of these restrictions are standard rules regarding informed consent and donation practices and are generally appropriate in any type of organ donation. The quirkiest limit, in the view of many, is a line in the sand drawn such that stem cell lines derived from blastocysts that were destroyed before August 9, 2001, are eligible to receive federal funding for research. Those stem cell lines derived from blastocysts destroyed after August 9, 2001, are not eligible for research with federal funds. This is the current policy.

It is a good, bad, and curious situation. In my view, the "good" (the bad in the view of some) is that some publicly funded research has started with hES cells, though not as vigorously as many of us would like. Even at the outset, many scientists had questions about the policy. Were all the stem cell lines of sufficient quality to support rigorous research? Would all the lines be "practically" available? (After all, some of the lines were held by private companies.) Would there be enough lines to support therapeutic application? Finally, the big one: If on August 10 additional excellent lines became available for research, what would happen then? This brings us to the "bad." We now know that the answer to the first three questions is a resounding "No." The outcome of this policy, if you fast-forward from 2001 to 2004, is that the sixty to eighty stem cell lines originally advertised by the administration as being available in 2001 and beyond have now been whittled down to nineteen available lines, according to the Web page of NIH. Anecdotally, it remains unclear whether some of the nineteen lines can actually be obtained by researchers. In addition, as I mentioned, there are substantial questions about the quality of these remaining lines. The "curious" aspect of the situation, of course, is that new lines of high quality have been obtained since August 9, 2001. These lines are being offered to the research community gratis as opposed to the $5,000 or so needed to purchase each federally approved line. These lines cannot be used with federal funds, or in facilities that have substantial federal funds being used in them, as is typical of most research laboratories in the United States.

It is likely that President Bush's policy will remain unchanged throughout his terms in office. A president has limited authority in deciding what the NIH can support. The president does not have the authority to decide that excess frozen IVF embryos held in freezers may be destroyed with public money. That would violate an ongoing annual amendment to the appropriations bill called the Dickey Amendment. All the president can do is to allow more lines to be used—if and only if they are derived with private funds. The likely outcome is that federal legislation will not change. To my knowledge, there is little will in Congress to dispense with the Dickey Amendment, which is actually at the root of all of these policies. Partisan politics and Senate procedures are likely to confound any effort to change this crucial amendment.

HOW THE SYNERGY OF THESE ISSUES AFFECTS RESEARCH

The outcome of the politics and policies regarding hES cells is an extremely complex research landscape. I will give you one example from my experience as a research scientist in California. In the next few months, I hope to have federal funding to do research with hES cells that are on the federally approved list. A month or two ago, a paper by Doug Melton at Harvard was published that reported the creation of seventeen new hES cell lines that are available and appear to be of very high quality. If I'm going to launch a multiyear research program with the public trust behind me, since even my private funds come from various sources of philanthropy, donations from people afflicted with disease and who would like to see cures, I have a number of important decisions to make as a research scientist about how I should proceed. When launching a multiyear program, first I need to compare these new cell lines and their properties to the older cell lines on which I may work using public dollars. I then must make a decision about what is going to be best for the research. Depending on the comparison, I may decide that I need to seek private funding for the endeavor. In the context of a typical research laboratory this becomes more complicated, since most American laboratories are supported by both public and private funding. It can be difficult to determine which dollars are spent where. For example, I would have to track and segregate all test tubes, reagents, and materials and in some cases account for electricity and other support services paid for with federal overhead. It would create a fairly significant bureaucratic oversight structure to ensure that I would use no public (federal) dollars on these cell lines derived a few months ago. Keeping a scientist from using federal dollars for research with these newer cell lines does not prevent any additional frozen blastocysts from being destroyed. These policies serve only to hinder research.

Unfortunately, it is unlikely that we will get a broad national consensus in the near future. In fact, a patchwork of state initiatives has developed in the absence of federal initiatives in this area.

THE (MIS)USE OF SCIENTIFIC INFORMATION

Progress is hindered by misunderstanding and, I think, blatant misuse of scientific information. Obviously, it is important to debate the ethical dimensions of research, but care must be taken to ensure that the ethical debate does not unduly influence the collection, interpretation, and evaluation of scientific data, which must be done as objectively and dispassionately as is humanly possible. It is critical that if scientific data are to be used to support or bolster a particular moral or ethical viewpoint, those data must be correct, accurate, and evaluated objectively.

How can scientific information be used responsibly in the policy debate that surrounds stem cell research? Some people believe that embryonic stem cells are going to solve everything; others think that adult stem cells are going to solve everything. Finally, most scientists in the field, as nearly as I can tell, are, like me, in the middle. We think we should pursue both avenues of research vigorously on the basis of the scientific data available thus far. Because of the media's attempt to give equal time to both sides of this scientific issue, the range of opinion has been portrayed by the media as indicating two distinct camps in the scientific community from which one must choose. Policy makers and people uncomfortable with the moral aspects of embryonic stem cell research also have portrayed potential breakthroughs in adult stem cell research as so promising that they obviate the need to confront the moral issues with embryonic stem cell research. Is this an appropriate policy argument, given what we know about the science?

EMBRYONIC "VERSUS" ADULT STEM CELLS

Work on the mouse, done over two decades, has established almost beyond the shadow of a doubt—which is as close as you can get in scientific research, for nothing can be proven with 100 percent certainty—that embryonic stem cells derived from blastocysts are pluripotent: that is, they can make every adult cell type. That is a principle, not a demonstration that you can cure a disease with them. It is an understanding of what their material properties are. The theoretical and experimental foundation for the notion that embryonic stem cells will aid in understanding and curing disease arises from this principle. In fact, in the mouse and, more recently, in the human there has been some progress in the fulfillment of these aims. With human cells, we aren't there yet. We are at the beginning of a research and development problem, not the middle or the end. Yet there are good proof-of-principle data that make most scientists optimistic that excellent understanding of disease and new approaches to treatment for terrible diseases are forthcoming over the next several years from hES research.

What do we know about adult stem cells? Cells from bone marrow, for example, are incredibly useful for the treatment of diseases of the blood and immune system. I would never say that we should not be working with these cells or using them in therapy or working to expand their uses. But if I am thinking about how to treat Parkinson's disease, these are not the first cells I am going to look at. Adult stem cells from bone marrow seem likely to have limited application, based on the data thus far. Most work to date suggests that adult stem cells have somewhat restricted potency. Although the biotechnology industry tried for close to a decade to grow bone marrow (hematopoetic) stem cells, the effort was a total failure as I understand it. Hundreds of millions of dollars were spent, and no one could devise a way to grow them efficiently. Though we may be able to tomorrow, it is simply not yet possible.

Some recent experiments suggest that cells from bone marrow and brain have more potential than originally thought. These experiments raise the possibility that maybe the dogma is wrong. After all, we find periodically as we learn more that dogma can be wrong. However, I will point out that usually the dogma is right in science, and often based on a significant amount of evidence. Thus "the voice in the wilderness" is more often wrong than it is right. When dissenting voices do prove correct, however, they receive wide publicity, and that is what people remember. Thus perhaps adult stem cells have more potential than we once thought on the basis of the last several decades of experiments.

From a scientist's perspective, however, many of the experiments that suggest an unprecedented potential of adult stem cells have not been reproduced by other scientists. That does not mean that these experiments are incorrect; it means that they have not yet been reproduced. However, my opinion is that the experimental design and assays employed in many of these studies are flawed. While this is not true of all the experiments, it is certainly true of some, and, unfortunately, most notably of some of the studies that have found their way to CNN in the evening.

Furthermore, most evaluations of the data by experts on adult stem cell research (many of whom have had their work cited by opponents of hES research as evidence that we should abandon work on embryonic stem cells) state that current scientific evidence "does not support the contention that adult stem cells can replace embryonic stem cells." From

Minnesota, Dr. Catherine Verfaille, one of Senator Brownback's favorite scientists, has reported research data on adult stem cells derived from bone marrow suggesting that these stem cells may prove incredibly useful, perhaps as pluripotent as embryonic stem cells. Yet Dr. Verfaille has stated publicly that it is too early to make a decision about which cell type is best and for which applications. We are simply not far enough down the path of research to know which cell types are going to be best for each potential use. In fact, Dr. Verfaille is running an institute that is trying to recruit researchers who work on embryonic stem cells, even though her own work is on adult stem cells.

If you consult other top U.S. researchers doing adult stem cell work, such as Dr. Irv Weissman, Dr. Fred Gage, or Dr. Sender, they will all tell you the same thing. Work on adult stem cells is certainly promising for some applications, but you cannot take the scientific data as justification for the argument that we shouldn't work on embryonic stem cells. Thus the debate about whether to use hES cells is purely a moral debate at this time. It is not appropriate to use the present scientific data to argue that we shouldn't proceed with hES cells for research and therapy development.

Given this controversy, I will close with a question that plagues the policy issue. What is the best approach when the scientific issues are not all settled? Is it appropriate to adopt a public policy, particularly a prohibitive public policy, in a situation where the data are not all in and where there is no decisive settlement of the moral and ethical debate? That is the policy issue in which we find ourselves and that we must confront in California and other states.

THE ROLE OF THE STATES IN SETTING POLICY

Are the states an appropriate venue for progress, given that the federal government is, in my view, stalled and likely to remain that way for some time? States are the "laboratories for experimentation" and allow more latitude for national disagreement. Some states can go one way, some can go another. The spectrum of solutions in this parallel system of experimentation leads inevitably, however, to the problem of a national patchwork in interstate commerce. On the other hand, the utilization of states as the venue for differing rules for hES research does allow scientific progress, albeit while maintaining some limits. Perhaps that's the best we're going to be able to do.

In California, the political debate is effectively over on this issue. Over the course of the past few years, several bills were passed and signed by the governor that allowed stem cell research of all sorts, established embryonic stem cell registries, began developing the regulatory framework for the research to proceed, and have come up with state funding. I do not foresee these California laws being changed because of apparently strong popular support among people in California. Moreover, states other than California—for example, New Jersey—have followed suit in validation of this approach. On the other hand, some states such as Arkansas have gone the other way. In California and New Jersey, there is the possibility of substantial state funding to make up for the federal shortfall. In some ways, California has unique positioning to take advantage of these technologies: we have the fifth largest economy in the world. We are bigger than most nations. We have anywhere from one-third to one-half of all the biotechnology companies in the United States, the greatest universities, and, I believe, the greatest scientists. California is thus uniquely positioned to have a large impact on the science, with consequent benefits for the California economy. Many of us think that the biotechnology part of the California economy is essential to the health of the state's economy and would not like to see it moving overseas to nations that invest more heavily in this area.

ADDENDUM: TWO FREQUENTLY ASKED QUESTIONS

Question 1 Who owns the intellectual property that results from stem cell research? And how does the public get return on its investment?

Answer 1 For federally funded research, because of the Bayh-Dole Act, intellectual property generated as a result of that funding belongs to the research institution that houses the investigator. The reason is that, prior to Bayh-Dole, when the government owned the intellectual property, the government did a poor job of getting the patent written, filed, and licensed to companies that would then develop the product. The patent is the beginning, not the end, of a licensing and development process. In my laboratory, when I patent things that I think will have benefit through development, the patent belongs to the University of California, jointly with the Howard Hughes Medical Institute because they pay my salary. Then it is up to the University of California and the Howard Hughes Medical Institute to find a licensee who will develop that patent.

The return on public investment is only sometimes captured as direct benefit back into the state or federal coffers. It is more often captured as economic activity and improvements in health care. There have been a number of economic studies in this area, but I will point to my favorite: a study by a joint committee of the U.S. House and the U.S. Senate, chaired by Connie Mac of Florida, a noted fiscal and social conservative. That panel concluded—and I believe this number has not been challenged—that if you look at society's return on the investment in medical research over the past several decades, it runs on the average of 25 to 40 percent annually. Is that likely to be captured in the California bond initiative? I am betting that, given California's enormous activity in the biotechnology and pharmaceutical industries, it will play out over time in this way. And that investment will be similar to the federal investment in the way that that return is generated.

Question 2   What do those who oppose the use of embryonic stem cells on moral or religious grounds suggest should be done with frozen embryos?

Answer 2   I cannot address this question because I do not share those beliefs. I think that the research should proceed. I will point out that, though the fact is often forgotten in this debate, research with tissue derived from aborted fetuses is legal, and you can use federal funds for it. There is a surprising inconsistency in the law. In this case, an act that, I think, many people probably find more objectionable is supported by federal funding, while another activity, namely human stem cell research, which, from my conversations with those who oppose both activities, is somewhat less offensive, is not allowed to receive public funding. But that may be creating shades of gray that don't really exist.

CHAPTER 6

Roots and Branches of the U.S. National Debate on Human Embryonic Stem Cell Research

Lee L. Zwanziger

I was asked to offer a view of the U.S. national debate about human embryonic stem cell research (hESCR) at a conference, organized by the editors of this volume, entitled "Stem Cells: Science, Ethics, and Politics in Dialogue." The conference took place in California, in the spring of 2004, surrounded by hot debate about Proposition 71. Proposition 71 was to provide funds through bonds for the California Institute for Regenerative Medicine, a state institute for stem cell research, especially research that would not be eligible for federal funding under the current federal policy. Other participants have commented on California's situation (see especially chapter 5). The debate about Proposition 71 has highlighted two themes important in the national debate, control and social consequences: that is, first, questions of the proper degree of public oversight of public funds versus oversight by experts in the relevant field and, second, the promise of societal and individual benefits versus concerns about societal and individual risks. Proposition 71 was passed in November of 2004, and several aspects of those same themes have since been reopened, in court as well as in the news.[1] Regarding the question of control of public action and public funds, discussions continue about public oversight and possible conflicting interests. Regarding potential outcomes, discussions address the likely speed of cures, expected financial returns to the state, and ownership of intellectual property developed with public funds. Legal and legislative actions are changing rapidly; therefore I have concentrated on themes that are less time sensitive, though of current import.

The context of our national hESCR discussion is not simply neutral. Promotion of hESCR funding, for example, may invoke the need for more scientific education as the root of the problem, suggesting that adequate knowledge of hESCR would ease or eliminate dissent. The implication is that there exists no real basis for moral disagreement, just ignorance of facts. This is a case of what has become known as the *deficit model* of public understanding of science, the idea that objections from the public to products or proposals involving science result from a deficit of knowledge or understanding, for which better education is obviously the needed response. Such an assumption alludes to many topics of importance, such as the nature and meaning of objectivity and convention in knowledge, as well as the roles and meaning of facts and values in science and public debate about science policy, leading to questions of what process might best facilitate democratization of policy deliberation consistent with specialized science. Much has been written about these topics, in political science, science policy, and both the social studies and the philosophy of science, that I will not be able to survey here. One of the aspects of the hESCR public discussion in the United States that has been most disturbing, but perhaps may finally be helpfully revealing, is how relatively little in evidence this current and previous work has been. Social and philosophical influences embedded in national institutions contribute to default political assumptions of the debate, but that seems to be overlooked in calls for sound science. I emphasize science institutions here because of their central establishment and strong effect on the terms of the debate; one branch of the discussion is located there. I also note a contrasting branch of discussion, perhaps less predominant but still vigorous, that urges caution about science and technology in society. Both these branches have roots, and the roots are philosophical positions about the topics under discussion.

Repeated volleying on the hESCR issue has not always been edifying with regard to science and ethics,[2] but it may suggest aspects of our U.S. science policy process that need further examination. I suggest that such examination may facilitate insight into the levels of reciprocal indignation and perhaps even point toward some strategies for tolerating pluralism. I start with some groundwork on science and technology in our society, proceeding next to education and advocacy for science in society. Then I discuss briefly two contrasting but fundamental principles of evaluating science and technology in society and their related assumptions or default positions. Finally I turn to persisting conflict in matters of policy for biotechnology, and I close with a wavering hope for tolerance of pluralism those matters.

SCIENCE, TECHNOLOGY, AND POLITICS

To start, I want to assert that science and technology are different from politics. By the word *science* I refer to a range of types of inquiry into the natural world that aim at discovering truths about the natural world. I used the word *assert* because here I am simply assuming the epistemological value of science (see Haack 2003 for a full account). By *technology* I refer to devices and processes designed by humans to accomplish some purpose in that world, a definition similar to, though perhaps more restricted than, that defended by Pitt (2000). These premises are so basic that it may seem strange to highlight them here; I do so to acknowledge the insufficiency of social factors to account for scientific understanding, even while emphasizing the insufficiency of scientific understanding to determine good policy. For the hESCR discussion, the relevance is that scientific understanding can inform public policy making but that good policy requires many other considerations as well, factors not trumped by science. That is another reason for emphasizing that science is a particular activity of inquiry: not all thought, indeed not all thoughtful rigorous reason, is *science* as we use the term today. Science requires recognition of what is not science to avoid collapsing from robust scientific inquiry into scientistic ideology, which we really must avoid. The question of what we can learn about biological development from stem cells of any sort is scientific. The question of whether we can develop commercially viable stem cell–based products is technological. But the question of whether to support any of these federally is a policy question, involving ethical and practical considerations of what we ought to do, and how and why. Scientific and political or more broadly social considerations are indeed entwined—but that makes it so much the more important to avoid a situation or even the appearance of a situation in which science (sound science, expert science, and so on) reduces in the end to power seeking by an interest group.

The reason behind the entwining of the scientific and the political is sometimes that it makes for expedient rhetoric, but there are historical grounds as well. To examine them, we have to go back further than the administration of President Bush, at least to Vannevar Bush. In 1945 Vannevar Bush, director of President Franklin D. Roosevelt's Office of Scientific Research and Development, submitted a report called *Science: The Endless Frontier* (Bush 1945). The general point of the report was that the federal government should continue in peacetime to fund basic research and not dismantle the government-based research institutions associated with wartime, though the institutions should be modified for peacetime purposes. The view in the report was that basic research should be federally supported because it was a good thing and because it would be good for the national economy and health. Basic research was thus defended as a good in itself and as a means for the government to promote other social goods. The report went on to make more specific recommendations, including the general plan for the design and operation of the federal civilian grant-making agencies supporting science. Thus already we have built into our governmental institutions the idea that basic research, specifically emphasizing here biomedical research, is good in itself and good for our national health and economy. More generally, we have built in the idea that science and technology are entwined with public, governmental functions, publicly supported, and for public goods. Finally, we have built in a generally optimistic view of the entwining of science and technology with social aims in government institutions (Mann 2001).

But is that really so bad? It is our history after all, and science *is* good. My point, however, is that this institutional foundation is not a neutral starting point for deliberation about supporting areas of scientific research. To say it is not neutral is not antiscience; rather, we should recognize that our national-level institutions for selecting and supporting science were conceived in response to a particular set of problems, initially military, and were characterized by an unstable combination of motives: the *insulation* of internally directed basic research from politics and the *application* of knowledge and invention. This combination of motives has continued into the present and is even richer, more complex, and significantly more unstable now than it was then, suggesting that it is perhaps time to reassess whether the science policy model we have inherited is the best approach to policy on publicly funded science today (see Sarewitz 2000).

SCIENCE, EDUCATION, AND ADVOCACY

Part of the tension between public participation and specialized expertise in science policy is that knowledge is crucial to good deliberation and to genuine participation in such a national discussion. For example, if persons opposed human cloning but did not realize that somatic cell nuclear transfer (SCNT) names a process of cloning, they might support research involving human SCNT—but ignorance of the science would prevent them from genuinely participating in the deliberation and from recognizing, and in some way resolving, the resulting contradictions in their own professed positions.[3] More knowledge may indeed dispel some disagreement that is simply mistaken. It need not result in concord, however, because not all disagreement about science policy is due to ignorance or fear about science. Rayner (2004) summarizes three versions of deficit models, all familiar from hESCR debates, that explain dissent as due to deficiencies in knowledge of scientific fact, in the understanding of scientific process, and/or in trust in scientists. Taken alone or together, these would be insufficient to explain dissent overall because dissent may spring from a concern not addressed by science. But just as reliance upon deficit models may be taken to intemperate lengths, so too may rejections of them: scientific knowledge remains important in public assessments of science (as recently redemonstrated by Sturgis and Allum 2004), even though it is not sufficient for policy deliberation.

While failing to understand the science certainly results in bad debate and can lead to bad policy, understanding the science is not sufficient to ensure wisdom in either. Scientific expertise literally defines a true elite with respect to scientific knowledge, but that criterion does not define an elite with respect to moral or other extrascientific questions of what we as a society ought to do or to fund. Education about the relevant science is thus a delicate matter. Experts have to educate, since to teach one does have to be knowledgeable—it is not true that "those who can, do, but those who can't, teach." But experts may become advocates, or may be perceived as advocates, further tangling science and politics and the credibility of each. For example, if education is to be credible, then the educator-spokespersons must strive to correct misunderstandings regardless of whether the error is likely to have a favorable or an unfavorable effect on political support for research funding.

Scientists are called on by professional and academic societies to engage in outreach and advocacy for research. For example, the executive director of the American Society for Cell Biology points out that federal funding is limited and that if no one advocates for biomedical research, then sooner or later other programs will get more of the funding (Marincola 2003). The author also notes that scientists may well be the most effective advocates for science funding. Recently the past president of the American Association for the Advancement of Science analyzed problems our society faces with regard to science, prescribing in part better communication by scientists with the public (Jackson 2005). Editors of journals—*Science*, for instance—have also weighed in on questions such as federal funding for hESCR and have called on scientists to support and promote the cause; probably one of the most overt statements was the announcement by the *New England Journal of Medicine* of its intent to encourage manuscripts on the topic.[4]

But what has *not* been discussed in most, if indeed any, of the calls for communication and outreach leading to advocacy is the delicate balance of the costs and benefits of advocacy success. Two ways of recognizing and assessing advocacy's effectiveness come readily to mind: most obviously, advocacy is effective when advocates get what they want from whoever is targeted; but at the same time, it is effective when political opponents regard the spokespersons in question *as* effective advocates. Now, what happens when a field of science or its spokespersons come to be recognized as effective in advocacy? They will be discounted as being just a few more political advocates! After all, if the spokespersons in a field already are seen to be serving as advocates, then they are likewise seen as liable to have made assumptions promoting their cause. But since science aims at understanding the natural world, that is a huge loss. It is a loss to us all because then no one can be trusted to tell the sometimes politically uncomfortable truth about some aspect of the natural world insofar as it is currently known, truth that might, for instance, cost a lot of money to address or for some other reason come as unwelcome news to a powerful constituency.

When scientists or science institutions choose to become political activists for any particular policy option in the name of science, they incur risks to the policy option and to the field of study. Recognizing and balancing the risks is delicate, much as in education. Of course, in the United States individuals, including scientists, enjoy the right to freedom of speech, including the right to advocate for a preferred policy option as well as to educate about the science (with respect to which multiple policy options can then be developed). But these are quite differently directed actions. When experts become identified with a political cause, their relation to it encourages opposing political activism accompanied by selection of complementary though more congenial experts. And this then guarantees further rounds of the same (punctuated intermittently with reciprocal claims of "But they started it!"). Identifying and advocating a particular policy option on grounds that the policy is uniquely scientific results in the policy disagreement being recast as a scientific disagreement. One result of that is to present alternative policy options as *unscientific* and to thereby promote insistence upon alternative scientific approaches for political reasons (Pielke 2004). This is not surprising because once an extrascientific difference is recast as "a scientific issue," the only point of entry to engage in the debate is likewise in scientific terms. But that recasting also implies that the issue (or at least all that is important about it) is a technical problem, solvable by experts. The political import of that implication is readily recognizable. In brief, short-circuiting the policy discussion in the name of sound science does not protect science; on the contrary, it tends to politicize science.

FEDERAL FUNDING AND ETHICS

The concrete expression of the hESCR debate in the United States is public funding because it determines which programs are federally controlled. The actual acts of manipulating, studying, modifying, or destroying in the course of research and development involving products starting with human embryos are not federally prohibited. The difference based on funding does not, of course, suggest that only the federally funded research is ethically important. It is sometimes suggested that this difference, in particular about hESCR, reflects direct moral hypocrisy or contradiction, as if the claim were that a particular act would be ethical if privately or state funded but would be unethical if federally funded.[5] This objection neglects the practical situation. It may be reasonable to hope that policy and law will be crafted in accord with morality, but it is not reasonable to expect this crafting to occur in isolation from precedent, tradition, current sentiment, and preexisting law. Federal funding is the concrete point that gives the federal government its regulatory foothold in connection to the issue.

The federal/private funding distinction serves further as a homely but effective safety valve for individual liberty in controversial practices, with a presumption of liberty. To the extent that the practices are construed as private matters, they may be left unhindered as private decisions. Construed as public actions, as they would be if publicly funded, they would be subject to public judgment. Thus the suggestion that the "general acceptance" of in vitro fertilization (IVF), which, as currently practiced in the United States, often results in nonimplanted embryos, is or ought to be a reason to fund hESCR more broadly (Cohen 2004) overlooks the practical situation that IVF is treated as a private medical decision. Persons who do not approve of the practice avoid it. If it were to be funded publicly, then it would need examination and assent not only from those who approve it but also from those who do not approve (whether it would meet general approval when approval was needed in concrete form is another question, and I don't know the answer). But for hESCR one can hardly leave the matter there, in part because the matter is research rather than case-by-case medical judgment. This raises questions, to which I now turn, of how federal funding of scientific research has come to be seen as an imperative (Callahan 2004) and why challenges to that assumption evoke such consternation.

BRANCHES OF THOUGHT ON SCIENCE AND SOCIETY EXPRESSED IN THE hESCR DEBATE

The Bush Report's View

While the Vannevar Bush report (1945) marks the inception or modification of civilian national science agencies, its entwining of science and social good in the state reflects ideals of optimism through Enlightenment-style approaches to the scientific and technical management of societal problems. So if this branch of the debate starts with the premise "Good science is good policy," then the related argument for social results is "If we do Research X (here, hESCR), then Societal Situation Y will follow" (where Y is something good, like curing serious diseases, so the research should be done, and not just by whatever means, but by funding from federal science agencies).

Is this a compelling argument for funding the research? It depends, of course, on the details. To the extent that the reason for doing hESCR is the socially valuable potential outcome of curing diseases, then it matters whether the particular research leads to cures and whether that path is the best, and the only, path to a cure for that medical problem. In general we cannot predict that with any certainty. And this brings up another way "it depends," namely that the general approach that funding basic research is good in itself and will also be good for the health and economy of the country gets general public assent just as long as there is general public agreement with the research in question (though general public agreement is perhaps unnecessary; rather, it is enough if there just is no stress or outcry due to strong *dis*agreement). Disagreement may arise because of something other than the outcomes claimed, such as the particular acts required in research, as in hESCR, or because of differing judgment of what outcomes are to be counted for consideration, or because of differing judgments about the allocation of scarce resources for supporting biomedical research and development. When there is such disagreement, it raises all sorts of questions about which projected outcomes are significantly likely, and which are desirable, but also about how that gets decided and who gets to decide. To frame the issue as if it were purely a matter of science, thus obviating or eliminating extrascientific concerns or questions raised by nonexperts as merely political interference, is no way to depoliticize the issue.

Several specific arguments that have been highlighted in the hESCR debate express this current of thought:

- We need more hESCR immediately to develop curative medical products without delay, but the research must be federally funded because any medical products are far too distant and uncertain for the research to attract sufficient private capital.

- Science is global or at least transnational, so if the research is not federally funded in the United States it will be done in other nations, which then will get "ahead" of the United States, with the corollary point that U.S. scientists may even relocate.

- Although concrete benefits in the form of medical products cannot be predicted with specificity in this or any other area of research, we must first do the research in order to know.

- Since the research raises ethical questions for many, it should be federally funded so it can be brought under federal regulatory oversight.

The first point illustrates the tension in arguing for basic research on the basis of applications and leads to questions such as: To the extent that our publicly funded research is justified as providing public benefits, ought we have greater institutional infrastructure for public determination of what is salient and how to proceed? How can we decide that hESCR rather than any other research path is the means to those benefits? And how are we to integrate public concern with the natural but limited scope of elite scientific expertise?

The second illustrates the tension between the presumed inevitability of the direction of science and technological development and the contingency of national history. It especially recalls our history in the model of national science policy shaped extensively by the World War II experience, in which the race to build the bomb became a wartime imperative and the national location of scientists was crucial. The national security race was also important later in science funding and the formation of policy supporting the space race. The implication of the second point is that hESCR is an international race that the United States must win at all costs.[6] To explore the points of similarity and difference in the situations is beyond the scope of this essay, but we cannot simply assume that the hot or cold wartime metaphors apply smoothly to hESCR or that the definitions of the runners, the race course, and the finish line are transferable.

The third and fourth points have much good sense—but only when seen in the limits of their initial context. Thus they illustrate the tension between, on the one hand, deliberating *whether and why* to engage in a particular research program and, on the other hand, simply passing over those questions to discuss *how* to do it. They can have little impact on those with the ethical doubts, however, since if someone seriously doubts whether something ought to be done at all, offering to fund it publicly to find out its particular consequences, or even to regulate how it will be done, cannot be considered any compromise on the "whether" question. Thus it is only to be expected that these points do not lay the issue to rest.

The design of the science agencies as institutions of government funding for research, however, was intended to keep the decisions about what is funded in the hands of scientists with expertise in the particular field, and also to insulate as much as possible from politics the process of allocating funds. This would include insulating the process from elected officials and thereby the general voting public. The degree to which publicly funded science would be under the control of elected officials (often not scientists), as opposed to scientific experts (not elected and therefore not necessarily accountable to taxpayers), was certainly a subject of debate at the time, just as it is now (Kevles 1977). So while Vannevar Bush believed, with good reason, that basic research would eventually lead to practical benefits, the institutional system that he envisioned for funding science was not designed to solve particular social problems identified by the general public as needed and desirable, or to facilitate dealing with subsequent events not intended or even anticipated but related to the research program (Sarewitz et al. 2004).

Further, the system of allocating funds by expert peer review does not contemplate how any moral or other extrascientific concerns might be expressed or accounted for in decisions to withhold or provide public funding for particular branches of research (nor what reasons, if any, might count as legitimate for discussing whether to do such research at all). It is a difficult question, and while proposals worthy of exploration, ranging from philosophical foundations (Kitcher 2001) to institutional implementation (Guston 2004), are being examined, it remains a problem because it involves introducing new parties directly into decision making. The idea of setting limits on research activities is in itself neither new nor opposed to science: for example, we limit what can be done with human research subjects. Where that particular condition is not generally agreed to apply—and many people do not regard human embryos as human subjects in a morally relevant sense—what can be the basis of discussion? Perhaps that situation accounts for the acrimonious tone of our national discussion of hESCR. Many of our fellow citizens do regard certain types of research as off limits for moral (hence extrascientific) reasons and suspect that their concerns will be dismissed as "unscientific" or "values" objections, while others see no reason to hesitate and do see desperate urgency to fulfill the promise of benefits.

The Critical View

Along with our "Good science is good policy" tradition, we have a smaller but also traditional branch of thought on the role(s) of science and technology in society, suggesting that caution about science and technology is good policy. This is a broad phenomenon, but in the United States social criticism of science and technology has often focused on environmental effects or information technology and privacy, and also, closer to the topic at hand, on what some see as the overmedicalization of areas of life like childbirth. This type of social criticism is often allied with and complemented by philosophies of technology, as in Langdon Winner's book *The Whale and the Reactor* (1986), where the author contrasts the fitting natural animal and the out-of-place nuclear reactor.

Just as the Bush (1945) branch of the debate on science in society reflects Enlightenment assumptions, this branch has historical roots supporting its twentieth-century expressions—here, from the Romantic period. In his account of attitudes toward technology, Mitcham (1994) discusses those mentioned here as "Enlightenment Optimism" and "Romantic Unease" and observes that for all the commentary generated by the latter attitude of caution, this current of thought has not produced as much concrete effect in societal action. Its relatively lesser effect may be due to many different conditions, including our institutional structures, but an additional factor may be the very formulation of the program. That is, the program is negative: don't move too fast, don't overlook the potential for unintended consequences, et cetera. One can be in sympathy with the various types of doubt and caution and still see that fewer positive recommendations for action must limit at least the observable effects. Nevertheless, its persistence in individual and small community practices shows that science and technology development can be accepted on terms other than the extremes like "inevitability" or "progress"—the latter in contrast to an image of a dark age.

Many of the topics or issues mentioned are associated, in the United States at least, with generally leftist politics (environmentalism, appropriate technology, feminism in reproductive health). Criticism of science and technology in society is an important current in many political sensibilities, however.[7] Recall, for instance, that in the national discussions on human cloning one of the big stories was how critics on both the left and the right were opposing cloning in very similar terms: for example, often invoking the potential instrumentalization of women or women's bodies or the potential commodification of ova.[8] This was politically remarkable, but it might be expected to occur for other issues of science and technology as well because "left" and "right" are not adequate proxies for thought and experience and thus cannot capture the common philosophical concerns. The argument of both urges that we not limit our discussion of science policy to questions of *how* (under the assumption that science and technology develop along some inevitable trajectory) but also consider *whether* we want to choose one direction, or avoid some other.

In arguments objecting to hESCR, a shared idea is that technology can be dangerous and can lead to bad consequences not limited to individual harms. The form of the argument contrasts with the "Good science is good policy" approach: "If we do Research X (here hESCR), then Societal Situation Y will follow" (where Y is something bad, like instrumentalization of women as egg donors or of human embryos as research material, so the research should not be done). Since that absolute recommendation is probably not an enforceable goal in the case of portable work such as hESCR, the argument may be at least that it should not be done in a particular state or that it should not receive public funding.

Is this a compelling argument against funding the research? Again, it depends, in some very similar ways to the science policy position mentioned. First, if the reason for not doing or not supporting an area of research is not the act itself but the prediction that the research will lead to bad social consequences, then we have to be clear on just what research leads to what consequences, and how we can be so sure that there is a causal link between the research and the projected consequences, and that there is no way other than blocking the research to avoid them. In practical terms one might avoid the research in one place, or even avoid it completely worldwide, and the undesirable outcome Y could still occur. That type of reasoning is called "denying the antecedent," and it is invalid precisely because the result might come about in another way even without the antecedent. The previous "Good science is good policy" argument supporting research funding for the sake of good social consequences is invalid in the same way: not doing or not funding the research does not guarantee that the desirable outcome, finding cures for serious diseases, would not occur through research other than hESCR. In the political discussion, however, either invalidity is admitted as a weakness only for the argument proposed by one's *opponents;* in fact both arguments proceed not by logical validity but by projections about the relative likelihood of uncertainties, with vivid assessments of the relative importance of the projected good and bad outcomes. And that brings up the second way that "it depends": it depends on agreement about what would count as a significant and likely social consequence, and that brings up all over again the questions about how it gets decided, by whom, and what counts as significant among the good or bad consequences.

LOCATING THE NATIONAL DEFAULT POSITION

If we considered hESCR merely as a branch of biology, the amount of attention at all levels of public life that has been devoted to it would be astounding and inexplicable. But the attention is more understandable in view of how it illustrates features of our past and present culture with respect to science and technology in society.

First, the hESCR debate has brought to the fore historic and contingent aspects of the relation of science and government, highlighting default assumptions about science in society. A default assumption need not be justified itself, but a suggestion of deviation does require justification. Default status confers great advantage and is thus desirable to keep or to obtain.

Second, what counts as justification in public debate must be publicly perceivable, concrete, and objective; hence moral concerns can be expressed in terms of harms to individuals on the model of research in human subjects, but many other types of moral concerns approaching notions of intrinsic worth are generally disallowed (Kaebnick 2000). As a result, we rely heavily on projected social costs and benefits (Lysaght et al. 2005). Cost-benefit analysis is rational and indispensable for deciding between different means for how to get to a given goal. It is not adequate, however, for deciding whether a particular goal ought to be selected in the first place.[9]

Third, the combination of which sorts of moral evaluations of science and technology are generally accepted as fair for public discussion and which sorts are disallowed (such as invocation of the sacred or values) drives the discussion, so that the debate takes place solely on scientific terms, on a linear model of science determining policy (Pielke 2004). As a result, proponents on either side must urge that their preferred policy option or preferred stem cell source should be favored because it will lead to the most effective medical interventions soonest. This argument must be driving the whole series of reports, claims, and counterclaims in a way that suggests scorekeeping with regard to numbers of potential treatments under investigation, or numbers and ranks of scientists endorsing hESCR or any alternatives. While the number of potential treatments is contentious in part because of different possible ways of counting, the number of scientist endorsers seems hardly relevant at all.[10] I have even had people ask me which kind of stem cell, embryonic or adult, is "better"—but better how and for what? If the question means better for developing cures—that is, biomedical products—then the answer may turn out to depend on the particular disease or condition and on the sort of technology we want to develop in order to cope with it. The question, however, shows that the idea of a generalized competition between stem cells for scientific and political status has been communicated and that the competition is couched in terms of which is a better problem-solving approach for medical product development—that is, in terms of projected outcomes, but only in those terms.

Casting the debate in terms of claims about relative magnitude or speed of producing hypothetical cures for diseases and conditions results in arguments over how to compare current research and future potential, provoking dueling claims of who is expressing scientific opinion or personal opinion. Meanwhile the number of persons potentially to be helped, 128 million, is quoted repeatedly and dates, as far as I can tell, from a Viewpoint essay in *Science* (Perry 2000). Such an estimate does not readily admit of refutation by experiment, but the iconic status that the number itself has assumed leads to reflection on a moral problem of instrumentalization at least as worrisome as the potential exploitation of women for ova, namely the instrumentalization of current as well as future potential patients and families by promised hope or even promised cures. In the context of moral argument about policy that is couched in terms of medical benefits to individuals, the promises of cures are just what we should expect, and caveats that clinical studies, let alone approved products, may be far in the future fade into insignificance even when they are included. It is a problem surely not limited to stem cell research (Schwartz et al. 2002), and it forms an important part of the context of this debate: if the argument for doing and/or funding research is driven by projections of biomedical products to be developed, then an outcome we can predict with high reliability is the touting of the promised benefit. That can range from expressions of genuine optimism to cynically calculated promotion mixed in any proportion, but while the argument is aimed at politicians, policy makers, and finally voters in general, it engages the hopes and hearts of patients.

In summary, we have a situation of rules (or at least expectations) of engagement, backed up by institutional history, tending to frame moral questions regarding hESCR so that they are subsumed under science and technology, best left to experts in the relevant scientific or technical area. In effect, this situation presumes that moral and any other extrascientific concerns are or at least ought to be ceded on the basis of scientific expertise. An alternative suggestion, that they be brought under a related institutional structure and formulation like our human research subject protection system and treated with bioethics expertise, reveals related problems.[11]

One illustration of the effects of national-level default status may be seen in the National Academies' reports on hESCR (National Research Council/Institute of Medicine [NRC/IOM] 2005), which recommend guidelines for voluntary compliance by all stem cell researchers regardless of their source of funding (and stem cells). As others have discussed (Robert and Baylis 2005), the panel, which recommended a model similar to the institutional review boards for human subjects protection, found few potential directions of hESCR to be problematic in themselves. Further, in the statement of task (NRC/IOM 2005, 3, 22), the panel emphasized that in this report they "did not revisit the debate about whether" hESCR should be done, assuming that it would be. The word *revisit* suggests that the issue had previously been addressed and may refer to a previous report on the scientific and medical aspects of hESCR (NRC/IOM 2001). But while that previous report repeats several times that there is deep division on the moral aspects of human embryo usage, it either emphasizes what might be the scientific benefit of pursuing it or refers the matter to future ethical discussion. The question of whether it ought to be done obviously received an implicit *yes* in the context: in other words, it was the default position (nor is this an isolated instance; see Maienschein 2003, 187).

The Academies' earlier report carefully noted that it was limited to scientific and medical aspects of stem cell research, so treating the reports as if they constituted a complete consideration would do both the Academies' panels and the topic a disservice. Worse, it can only confirm the suspicion of persons who fear that their moral concerns will be overwhelmed by the presumption that the disputed developments in science and technology are inevitable. My point here is not to argue about what the Academies panels should have been doing in 2001 or in 2005—they answered their charge as requested by the parent institution and any external funders. But science and ethics-of-science advisory bodies are often asked to deliberate extrascientific questions where the formulation of those questions is highly constrained, given that they are boundary organizations in the context of an established default position on moral questions related to science and technology.[12] Thus while a particular report, here the NRC/IOM 2005 report, can help demonstrate this, we must recognize that the problem is broader than the charge of the particular panel.

LOCATING THE NATIONAL FAULT LINES

Arguments about what we ought to do publicly regarding hESCR start from some (usually tacit) idea of the thing talked about and its basic nature, which then influence attitudes regarding where or by whom further decisions should be made. The "idea of the thing talked about" may be the embryo (or pre-embryo) itself, or it may be the entire human life cycle (from biological procreation through growth through procreation of the next generation). What exactly is the important thing being changed? Has it a basic nature at all, and does it have moral standing, symbolic value (only), or material function (only)? Obviously these are not mutually exclusive categories, but that is just one more complication. The potential medical benefits of hESCR may well cause everyone to agree that such results would be desirable, but they will have no effect whatever on people's position about whether human embryos are the sort of thing to be available for that use. Protecting vulnerable developing human life may be something everyone wants, but agreeing on that has no effect at all on the position of whether in vitro human embryos are the sort of thing to be protected. Thus the debate also points to fault lines in our points of view. For example: suppose one starts thinking about whether we should fund hESCR with a fundamental idea that a human individual is *(a)* autonomous, characterized by capacities gradually emergent from the developing body, or in contrast, *(b)* intrinsically involved in network of relationships, at least some of which precede the individual body's development. Indeed, many of our differences are located at the level of ideas of what the thing (here the human thing) really and most basically is, underlying whatever else we think or know or observe about it. And there are also other deep-level discords, such as whether goodness exists or whether it is a matter of convention. Intractability of disputes at this basic level does not itself imply that no truth exists in moral matters, but it does suggest that we are unlikely to settle it by national consensus.

Persons in accord on matters such as either *(a)* or *(b)* above develop compelling ethical reasoning for what ought to be done. But if they are not in accord (if some hold position *(a)* and some hold position *(b)*), they will need time and goodwill even to understand what the other is talking about. Without that effort, the position that follows from one type of initial view will appear absurd to the other, but denouncing one's opponent by *reductio* to a position that is absurd only relative to premises that the opponent does not hold in the first place demonstrates only one's own lack of penetration.

One could formulate this fault line in many ways: viewing human nature as malleable by human design or as mainly stable; viewing human mortality as a problem (to be solved) or as a condition (to be accepted); and of course viewing moral standing as gradually emerging as a result of developing capacities or as a result of instantiating a kind of being that has moral standing. It is important to note that these paired alternatives not only suggest a fault line between positions but also highlight certain dimensions of the dispute. Other pairs, such as viewing a woman as someone who experiences much of adult life as potentially fertile and potentially a mother versus viewing a woman as someone who is potentially an egg donor responsive to superovulatory stimulus, would highlight different, though still related, dimensions. But any given pair provides only a partial view; thus focusing on any one of these examples necessarily screens off consideration of different but not necessarily opposed aspects of the question. Though inadequate descriptors, they nevertheless are valuable as reminders that if participants in the hESCR debate lack insight into the roots of their own position, they are unlikely to be able to discuss it with others whose positions are differently rooted. The political positions people take, whatever these may be, reflect not only how they judge their or anyone's *interests* likely to be best served by projected, as yet unrealized, social consequences but also what they take to be the actual *nature* of the object under discussion, whether "the embryo," "human nature," or even "nature" ("the environment") or "science." I am quite sure many readers have by now heard that it is only an irrational misunderstanding or cruel disregard for human life that leads some of us to be willing to grant public funding to research that destroys human embryos in the hope of developing new medical products. Likewise, many readers must by now have heard that it is just an irrational misunderstanding or cruel disregard for human life that leads others of us to call for only nonembryonic source of cells for research in treatment for terrible diseases or to withhold public funds for that research. Neither statement captures our situation, and although accusations in both directions will no doubt continue to be made, that approach is not getting us anywhere and is not going to get us anywhere.

CONCLUSION

This view of U.S. national debate about hESCR shows several obvious features:

- Science agencies and science policy making have institutionalized the "Good science is good policy" approach: the idea that good science is determined by expert scientists, with a view to applications.
- Thus there is at least a pro-research default position, if not a research imperative.
- Advocacy on both sides is cast in terms of sound science in general and selected outcomes in particular.
- Science agencies at the national level have the ability to fund or not fund, and so to exercise control over research activity only by first endorsing it.
- Meanwhile, balancing institutions and practices (here, the Congress) for considering different or additional selection criteria are not similarly specialized but must have many unrelated priorities.

These points are not the premises of an argument but descriptions of a context strongly inclined to favor science and technology, and as a result, to favor the formulation of moral and other extrascientific questions in terms of science, thus bringing them likewise into line with the context. Nevertheless, the context includes another feature:

- Resistance to the default position persists.

Despite the loneliness of the last little point, it survives. That is why we have a national debate, because of individual resistance to reframing moral questions as scientific problems. It is not hard to see that we have a pluralistic society, though the hESCR issue demonstrates substantial reluctance to recognize, let alone tolerate, that diversity in practice. Debate about hESCR, so often in terms that are incommensurable rather than in direct opposition, illustrates what happens in the absence of any commonly acknowledged basis of morality and knowledge: "The Enlightenment hope of secular bioethics has gone aground on the postmodern recognition of competing moral narratives and accounts, among which choice in a principled fashion has not proved possible without begging the question of which moral vision should give guidance" (Engelhardt 2002, 10). A shared metaphysical (and moral and epistemic) grounding of any type would ease that tension. The strategy of restricting discussion, whether specifically in bioethics or in a general public forum, to what is not only secular and public but scientific may seem at first to offer a way to resolve or simply avoid this intractable problem. Needless to say, it does not succeed, because the project starts by defining terms (*human, embryo, moral, reasonable, progress*, etc.) in such a way as to beg the question just as Engelhardt describes.[13]

To the extent that our institutions, whether explicitly or by practical effect, result in national conformity, they impose a zero-sum, winner-take-all condition on the issues they govern. In particular, consider our public institutions for supporting science when the research program involves extrascientific concerns, as is the case with hESCR: first, the zero-sum, winner-take-all effect of national-level policy decisions results in a national debate with parties working to vanquish their opponents. And as an immediate result, even if compromises of regulation are suggested in good faith, they come with the implication of that same zero-sum accounting, so that a committed dissenter has nothing to lose by refusing compromise as long as any means of expression remains. To the extent that our national discussion depends on identifying a vision as if it were a neutral ground for compromise, no reasonable end is in sight.

Consensus models have the attraction of some degree of apparent inclusion, but that can be deceptive, masking actual divisions overlooked because the space at the table is limited for whatever reason.[14] In the face of such differences, the options include[15]

- Persuasion or conversion of opponents to concordant views. This involves providing specification for arguments: what the research really is, what effects it might have, and so forth. It may work, but rarely if persons are committed to any deep view.

- Coercion—this need not be illegitimate, as when enshrined in majority rule. It is, however, simply a ruling for one view to prevail and should be expected to be regarded as coercion by whoever "loses."

- Agreement on procedures and institutional structures permitting policy differences reflective of the deep ethical differences previously mentioned.

With respect to policy on science and/or medicine affecting uses of human embryos, we have been pursuing all three options, including agreement sought through national-level consensus committees, despite their problems. The "agreement" approach could be pursued through a more pluralistic federalism (hardly a new idea but a radical departure from recent expectations), with the idea that differing policies would be acceptable, and indeed more acceptable than enforced uniformity. Engelhardt (2002), Evans (2006), and Trotter (2006) all have argued in various degrees that our approach should attempt to address, rather than ignore or suppress, persistent pluralism. As is also true of Kitcher (2001), these arguments are far from implementable procedures and institutions (see Brown 2004). But they are far beyond the continued defense of consensus among selected expert participants in advisory committees and policy making that we have been treated to in the course of the hESCR debate so far. Thus even those who oppose hESCR uses of human embryos might appreciate the decision of a state such as California to support such research, with the implication that other states may choose to avoid it.

On a practical level, however, this last approach is both difficult and expensive for enterprises like interstate or even international science and commerce. It is in general increasingly uncommon in the United States, since more and more issues are dealt with at the national level and since many states may have little practical or economic ability to make an effective stand. One has only to note how often we invoke inconvenience as a reason for insisting on national uniformity while we respond to the acknowledgment of any real differences between people in different places by disparagingly describing those differences as "a patchwork." The pluralistic approach is difficult to support for another reason as well, namely that it requires that on issues of critical import (and if hESCR does not meet that criterion for you, there are many other candidates!) probably all of us must incur difficulty and expense for the sake of the deep commitments of opponents that seem to us to lack any real meaning or even to be clearly wrong. As a result I for one am not confident that pluralism will be long lasting on this issue. Nevertheless, by revealing and reemphasizing the roots and branching implications of decision making where viewpoints conflict in science and policy, the hESCR debate may provide impetus toward developing and implementing structures to accommodate difference; such at least is my hope.

NOTES

The author is employed as a staff member for the Food and Drug Administration's Drug Safety Oversight Board and as a visiting assistant professor of science and technology studies by Virginia Polytechnic Institute and State University. The opinions expressed here are the author's and may not reflect those of any current or previous employers. The author acknowledges helpful discussion and support from Jane Maienschein and the Center for Biology and Society at Arizona State University; helpful comments from (in alphabetical order) Rachel Ankeny, Jessica Bolker, Jane Maienschein, Lynette Reid, Jason Robert, and Mary Sunderland in a working meeting sponsored by the Model Systems Strategic Research Network (funded by the Stem Cell Network in Canada); and helpful comments from Philip Nickel and the other speakers at the conference from which this volume grew, the conference organizers and editors of this volume, K. Monroe and R. Miller, and two anonymous referees.

1. See, for example, Pollack (2005) and, for further analysis, Sarewitz (2006).

2. For consistency I have tried to follow the usage of *morals* and *ethics* laid out by Ronald B. Miller in chapter 8 of this book.

3. Similar terminological changes have been offered for *embryo* and *pre-embryo* to highlight the time of implantation (Danforth and Neaves 2005). Whether this change does indeed help to increase understanding and whether increased understanding helps one or the other political side are empirical questions beyond my scope. Still more radical changes have been reported (Holden 2006), suggesting that terminological specificity may have been recognized as detrimental to legislation in some contexts. Clearly, intentional obfuscation at least raises moral questions, but it is also true that in many such cases of an allegedly simple fact one must acknowledge that what appears as clarity or obfuscation depends on the context of the term or statement. With regret, given its relevance, I cannot pursue that topic here.

4. For example, see Kennedy (2003, 2004); "Turn of the Tide" (2004); and Drazen (2003). Obviously these samples do not even begin to capture the plethora of commentaries on the issue. This partial list is further limited to formal editorials, not letters to the editor or contributed individual perspectives.

5. See, for example, Cohen (2004) for a summary of these arguments. A similar claim is sometimes made about the date of President Bush's policy announcement, but I will not pursue that here.

6. Thus the assessment of the situation of scientific misconduct discovered in Professor Hwang's lab—"The race is back on, and I think the U.S. has a second chance to do it right"—was perhaps only to be expected (Dr. Robert Lanza, president of Advanced Cell Technologies, quoted in Weise 2006).

7. Examples could be numerous, but a recent issue of the *Hedgehog Review* (vol. 4, no. 3 [2002]) illustrates the point, including articles by Winner, A. Borgman, L. Andrews, and G. Meilaender and an interview with F. Fukuyama.

8. For just one example, see Abate (2001). For additional insight into the coalition on cloning and commodification, see online companion content to ch. 25, "Emerging Biotechnology: Cloning," in *Our Bodies Ourselves* (Our Bodies Ourselves 2005).

9. It may appear adequate if we have already identified the standard for comparison with respect to which we assess costs and benefits, pains and pleasures, and of whom or what. But that would assume we had already done what is still unsettled and contested in the hESCR case. If it could be simply done, we would not be having this acrimonious debate.

10. Actually, one organization has directly used the scoreboard metaphor to highlight the benefits of clinically oriented nonembryonic versus embryonic stem cell research (see the scoreboard pictured on the home page of the Coalition of Americans for Research Ethics at www.stemcellresearch.org, accessed May 3, 2007). It has been attacked on the basis of counting methods and endorsements (Smith et al. 2006), with responses to those critics appearing as this is being written (Prentice and Tarne 2007; for earlier additional discussion, see Orive et al. 2003; Orkin and Morrison 2002).

11. Evans (2006) analyzes the function or aspirations of public bioethics practitioners, commentators, and committees as a branch of technocrats. He does not take up the special case of hESCR, but the possible application is clear.

12. Boundary organizations, as the name suggests, are located between science and nonscience entities that make and execute policy—for example, science advisory committees and institutions. Boundary organizations "exist at the frontier of the two relatively different social worlds of politics and science, but they have distinct lines of accountability to each" (Guston 2001, 401). For an analysis of bioethics committees as boundary organizations, see Kelly (2003).

13. I need hardly point out that an effective ban (on research, not on a funding source) would be likely to invoke a similarly begged question. I did not focus on that alternative because it is not a practical possibility.

14. The application of consensus models in advice to the government, both technical and nontechnical, through the mechanism of scientific and bioethics advisory committees is an area of great personal interest and one that has inspired considerable comment, but it cannot be pursued here. One can hardly miss the observation that a committee of any workable size must either be selected in such a way to be able to come to consensus and thus leave out some positions (see Green 2001), or the opposite, in which case consensus is not to be expected (as seen in the President's Council on Bioethics).

15. The description here of intractable differences and the range of possible responses are greatly influenced by the ethical writings of H. T. Engelhardt; see, for example, Engelhardt (1999; 1996, esp. 67–72).

REFERENCES

Abate, T.
    2001. "Odd-Couple Pairing in U.S. Cloning Debate: Abortion-Rights Activists Join GOP Conservatives." *San Francisco Chronicle,* Aug. 8, A-1.

Brown, M. B.
    2004. "The Political Philosophy of Science Policy." *Minerva* 42:77–95.

Bush, V.
    1945. *Science: The Endless Frontier.* www.nsf.gov/od/lpa/nsf50/vbush1945.htm. Accessed Jan. 12, 2007.

Callahan, D.
    2004. "When Science Is Just Another Good Cause." *New Scientist* 181 (2436): 18–19.

Cohen, C. B.
    2004. "Stem Cell Research in the U.S. after the President's Speech of August 2001." *Kennedy Institute of Ethics Journal* 14 (1): 97–114.

Danforth, W. H., and W. G. Neaves.
    2005. "Using Words Carefully." Letter. *Science* 309: 1815–16.

Drazen, J. M.
    2003. "Legislative Myopia on Stem Cells." Editorial. *New England Journal of Medicine* 349 (3): 300.

Engelhardt, H. T.
    1996. *The Foundations of Bioethics.* 2nd ed. New York: Oxford University Press.
    1999. "Bioethics in the Third Millennium: Some Critical Anticipations." *Kennedy Institute of Ethics Journal* 9 (3): 225–43.
    2002. "Consensus Formation: The Creation of an Ideology." *Cambridge Quarterly of Healthcare Ethics* 11:7–16.

Evans, J. H.
    2006. "Between Technology and Democratic Legitimation: A Proposed Compromise Position for a Common Morality Public Bioethics." *Journal of Medicine and Philosophy* 31:213–34.

Green, R. M.
    2001. *The Human Embryo Research Debates: Bioethics in the Vortex of Controversy.* New York: Oxford University Press.

Guston, D.
    2001. "Boundary Organizations in Environmental Policy and Science: An Introduction." *Science, Technology, and Human Values* 26 (4): 399–408.
    2004. "Forget Politicizing Science. Let's Democratize Science!" *Issues in Science and Technology,* Fall, 25–28.

Haack, S.
    2003. *Defending Science—Within Reason: Between Scientism and Cynicism.* Amherst, NY: Prometheus Books.

Holden, C.
    2006. "Maryland Goes for Stem Cells." Science Scope. *Science* 312:35.

Jackson, S. A.
    2005. "The Nexus: Where Science Meets Society." *Science* 310:1634–39.

Kaebnick, G. E.
    2000. "On the Sanctity of Nature." *Hastings Center Report* 30 (5): 16–23.

Kelly, S. E.
    2003. "Public Bioethics and Publics: Consensus, Boundaries, and Participation in Biomedical Science Policy." *Science, Technology and Human Values* 28 (3): 339–64.

Kennedy, D.
    2003. "Stem Cells: Still Here, Still Waiting." Editorial. *Science* 300 (May 9): 865.
    2004. "Stem Cells, Redux." Editorial. *Science* 303 (Mar. 12): 1581.

Kevles, D. J.
    1977. "The National Science Foundation and the Debate over Postwar Research Policy, 1942–1945: A Political Interpretation of *Science—The Endless Frontier*." *Isis* 68:5–26.

Kitcher, P.
    2001. *Science, Truth and Democracy.* Oxford: Oxford University Press.

Lysaght, T., R. A. Ankeny, and I. Kerridge.
    2006. "The Scope of Public Discourse Surrounding Proposition 71: Looking beyond the Moral Status of the Embryo." *Bioethical Inquiry* 3:109–19.

Maienschein, J.
    2003. *Whose View of Life? Embryos, Cloning and Stem Cells.* Cambridge, MA: Harvard University Press.

Mann, A. K.
    2001. *For Better or Worse: The Marriage of Science and Government in the United States.* New York: Columbia University Press.

Marincola, E.
    2003. "Research Advocacy: Why Every Scientist Should Participate." *Public Library of Science Biology* 1 (3): 331–33. http://biology.plosjournals.org. Accessed Jan. 12, 2007.

Mitcham, C.
    1994. "Epilogue: Three Ways of Being-with Technology." In *Thinking through Technology: The Path between Engineering and Philosophy,* 275–99. Chicago: University of Chicago Press.

National Research Council/Institute of Medicine.
    2001. *Stem Cell Research and the Future of Regenerative Medicine.* Washington, DC: National Academies Press.
    2005. *Guidelines for Human Embryonic Stem Cell Research.* Washington, DC: National Academies Press.

Orive, G., et al.
    2003. "Controversies over Stem Cell Research." *Trends in Biotechnology* 21 (3): 109–12.

Orkin, S. H., and J. J. Morrison.
    2002. "Stem-cell Competition," *Nature* 418 (July 4): 25–27.
    Our Bodies Ourselves. (2005). "Assisted Reproduction, Companion Content,
        Emerging Biotechnologies: Cloning." Ch. 25. *Our Bodies, Ourselves*
        Companion Site. www.ourbodiesourselves.org/sitemap.asp. Accessed
        Jan. 8, 2007.

Perry, D.
    2000. "Patients' Voices: The Powerful Sound in the Stem Cell Debate."
        Science 287:1423.

Pielke, R. A.
    2004. "When Scientists Politicize Science: Making Sense of the Controversy
        over *The Skeptical Environmentalist.*" *Environmental Science and Policy*
        7:405–17.

Pitt, J.
    2000. *Thinking about Technology: Foundations of the Philosophy of
        Technology.* New York: Seven Bridges Press.

Pollack, A.
    2005. "California's Stem Cell Program Is Hobbled but Staying the Course."
        New York Times, Dec. 10.

Prentice, D. A., and G. Tarne.
    2007. "Treating Diseases with Adult Stem Cells." Letter. *Science* 315 (Jan.
        19): 328.

Rayner, S.
    2004. "The Novelty Trap: Why Does Institutional Learning about New
        Technologies Seem So Difficult?" *Industry and Higher Education* 18 (6):
        349–55.

Robert, J. S., and F. Baylis.
    2005. "Stem Cell Politics: The NAS Prohibitions Pack More Bark Than Bite."
        Hastings Center Report 35 (6): 15–16.

Sarewitz, D.
    2000. "Human Well-Being and Federal Science: What's the Connection?"
        In *Science, Technology, and Democracy,* ed. D. L. Kleinman, 87–102.
        Albany: SUNY Press.
    2006. "Proposition 71: Vulgar Democracy in Action." Presentation at the annual
        meeting of the American Association for the Advancement of Science, Feb.
        17, Symposium on Stems Cells and Society: Assessing a Grand Challenge,
        St. Louis, MO. www.cspo.org/ourlibrary/author/. Accessed July 27, 2006.

Sarewitz, D., G. Foladori, N. Invernizi, and M. S. Garfinkel.
    2004. "Science Policy in Its Social Context." *Philosophy Today* 48 (suppl):
        67–83.

Schwartz, L. M., S. Woloshin, and L. Baczek.
    2002. "Media Coverage of Scientific Meetings: Too Much, Too Soon?"
        Journal of the American Medical Association 287:2859–63.

Smith, S., W. Neaves, and S. Teitelbaum.
2006. "Adult Stem Cell Treatments for Diseases?" Letter. *Science* 313 (July 28): 439.

Sturgis, P., and N. Allum.
2004. "Science in Society: Re-evaluating the Deficit Model of Public Attitudes." *Public Understanding of Science* 13:55–74.

Trotter, G.
2006. "Bioethics and Deliberative Democracy: Five Warnings from Hobbes." *Journal of Medicine and Philosophy* 31:235–50.

"Turn of the Tide."
2004. Editorial. *Nature Medicine* 10 (4): 317.

Weise, E.,
2006. "Cloning Race Is on Again." *USA Today,* Jan. 17.

Winner, L.
1986. *The Whale and the Reactor: A Search for Limits in an Age of High Technology.* Chicago: University of Chicago Press.

CHAPTER 7

Stem Cell Politics: The Perfect Is the Enemy of the Good

Sidney H. Golub

My first real-life exposure to the aphorism, sometimes attributed to Voltaire, that the perfect is the enemy of the good occurred soon after my arrival in the national capital area in 1999. I was the newly appointed Executive Director of FASEB (Federation of American Societies for Experimental Biology), and I was undergoing my education by immersion into the politics of "advocacy." Veteran Washingtonians explained to me that becoming too enamored with the perfect solution to a problem was one of the most common pitfalls for a political process that functions best when common ground can be found among divergent political perspectives. For example, support of basic science research can be justified on humanitarian or economic development grounds, and both justifications result in the same desirable outcome. Those who insist on soliciting support based solely on the justification that it is the right thing to do may miss a chance for a productive alliance with those who see medical research as an economic issue. It is frustrating to those of us who see embryonic stem cells (ESCs) as a great scientific opportunity that the politics that govern stem cell policy have focused on absolutist outcomes and that compromise has found little appreciable political traction. There are some hopeful recent signs that this may be changing, but even if political positions become less entrenched, scientific opportunities have already been lost.

This commentary is intended to be a brief summary of the current status of the three areas where the politics of human ESCs plays out—federal policy, international policy and the policies of individual states.

FEDERAL POLICY AND LEGISLATION

Developing public policy regarding research that involves fetal or embryonic materials must navigate between the antiabortion sentiment that is so powerful in Congress and the equally powerful desire to support medical research. Medical research has enjoyed a long history of generous national support in the United States, and the 1998–2003 doubling of the National Institutes of Health (NIH) budget to approximately $28 billion was a clear statement that health research is a high national priority. Simultaneously, abortion policy has been the focus of much legislative and legal action over the past four decades. The tension that occasionally arises between these two issues resulted in a two-pronged national strategy, with research support allowed for already existing embryonic materials but prohibited for the development of new derivatives from embryos or fetuses. This sort of "legal fiction" allowed the government to take the position that nothing was being done to create incentives for abortion while still finding means to support promising avenues of medical research using these same materials. Investigators were required to find nonfederal support to obtain the materials but thereafter were eligible for peer-reviewed federal funding. Especially relevant in this policy was the NIH Revitalization Act of 1993, which permitted the use of fetal materials for transplantation (e.g., for Parkinson's disease) so long as they were obtained under strict guidelines.[1] This permissive policy was soon thereafter coupled with the annually renewed amendment to the NIH appropriation (the Dickey-Wicker Amendment) that prohibits the use of federal funds for the creation of embryos for research.[2] While not overtly in conflict, the divergent thrust of these two policies was in keeping with the separation of obtainment from use. This policy construct clearly influenced a draft policy being vetted within the NIH during the last months of the Clinton administration that followed the same general pattern for human ESCs by permitting federal funding for research but not for the establishment of new cell lines.

   The focus of federal human ESC policy in the recent past has been the "compromise" promulgated by President George W. Bush on August 9, 2001.[3] That policy allowed federal funding for research employing then already existing ESCs that met stringent ethical standards of informed consent and noncoercion. The unique feature of the August 2001 Bush policy was that the date of its promulgation, rather than some ethical standard, became a bright dividing line. Cell lines developed after that point could not be eligible for federal research funding. No new cell lines, including those established with nonfederal resources under the most stringent ethical guidelines, could ever become eligible for use in federally funding research projects. The logic of this policy is obviously strained; instead of adopting the usual formulation that if the government hands did not touch the establishment of the materials then its hands are clean, the new position is that once the government became aware that research was going on it could no longer countenance it. This is a major departure from past policy, and in retrospect it is apparent that the Bush policy simply deferred the debate to a later date. This policy would have been effective only if stem cells had proven to be a research dead end, but scientific success in ESC research guaranteed demands to reconsider this approach. Unfortunately, the Bush compromise of 2001 was the last effort at compromise to enjoy any support from the opponents of stem cell research.

NIH director Elias Zerhouni and others have maintained that the Bush policy is guided by the president's moral convictions.[4] This is in all likelihood quite true, but the policy was also clever short-term politics, since it positioned the president as nominally in support of stem cell research while not alienating the vocal and activist right-to-life elements of the electorate. The Bush compromise initially met with mixed reactions from the scientific and patient communities. While almost all the organizations representing scientists wanted greater latitude for ESC research, some viewed the Bush policy as a limited opportunity to use federal support to start "proof of principle" experiments to better determine the potential of stem cells.[5] Others doubted that the number of existing ESC cell lines was sufficient to carry even that limited burden.[6] As the number of readily available cell lines dwindled to its current twenty-one, advocacy organizations representing patients and scientists increased the pressure to relax the pre–August 2001 limitation on cell lines eligible for funding.

The 2004 presidential campaign made legislation or policy change unlikely in 2003–4. Stem cell policy was one of the rare science policy issues that actually made it into the broad political arena, as exemplified by a cover story in *Newsweek* (October 25, 2004). However, not even the appearance of former President Reagan's son Ron at the Democratic National Convention or polls showing wide support for modification of the Bush policy seemed to have much impact, as other issues dominated the campaign.[7] Following the reelection of President Bush, expectations were low for liberalization of federal stem cell policy via either new legislation or administrative action. Yet the issue of federal support for human ESC research has reemerged in 2005 with powerful bipartisan support. This renewal of interest in expanding ESC research is largely due to the persistence and effectiveness of patient advocacy groups with support from some of the nation's most eminent scientific leaders.

Opposition to expanded human ESC research includes many "prolife" or "antiabortion" legislators, and the argument against this research coalesces around the strong belief that an embryo should have the same legal status as a person. This viewpoint is well illustrated by a statement from the Web site of Senator Sam Brownback (R-KS): "Clearly, we must to continue to work to find cures for diseases, and to alleviate suffering. However, it has never been acceptable to deliberately kill one innocent human being in order to help another. Life begins at the beginning at conception. Human beings develop from the one-celled stage onward, and deserve respect because of the dignity they have as human beings."[8] This construct does not easily accommodate to legislative compromise, and its advocates have resisted any expansion of federal support for ESC research. One consequence of this rigid position is that the anti-ESC legislators have distanced themselves from the reality of how ESC research was going to be conducted so that the regulations that would be established for the use of human ESCs would be written by those who were already committed to the expansion of ESC research. This may be appropriate, but one wonders if there might not have been a broader consensus on the issue if there had been real engagement on the concept of how to actually use human ESCs.

It is important to recognize that there is not a complete coincidence of antiabortion and anti-ESC viewpoints, as many legislators who identify themselves as "prolife" are also vocal supporters of human ESC research. Stephen S. Hall, in his book *Merchants of Immortality,* describes in vivid detail the moving and influential testimony in 2001 by Senator Gordon Smith (R-OR).[9] Senator Smith's comments encapsulate the argument for federal support: "For me, being pro-life means helping the living as well. I choose to err on the side of hope, healing, and health. And I believe the federal government should play a role in research to assure transparency, to assure morality, to assure humanity, and to provide the ethical limits and moral boundaries which are important to this issue. . . . We are at the confluence between science and theology. I believe we must err on the side of the broadest interpretations to do the greatest amount of good." Senator Smith is one of the few politicians who has reached out to the opponents of ESC research with arguments based on mutually shared religious views of the sanctity of life. The "pro-life" proponents of ESC research are likely to be central in this political divide.

The brightest moment thus far for advocates of federal ESC support came on May 24, 2005, as the House of Representatives passed HR 810, as proposed by Representative Castle (R-DE) and Representative DeGette (D-CO), by a vote of 238–194.[10] This legislation would simply remove the August 9, 2001, limitation on the cells lines eligible for federal funding and would thereby expand eligibility beyond the current twenty-one cell lines. Given the support for anticloning legislation (discussed below) in the House, passage of HR 810 is a remarkable change in legislative approach. While the fate of this legislation in the Senate is uncertain and President Bush has promised a veto even if it is passed, the successful passage of HR 810 indicates growing political support for ESC research. It is notable that fifty Republican representatives supported this measure despite overt opposition from the White House. One possible cause for this shift is the passage of Proposition 71 in California and the subsequent move among a number of states to provide local resources for ESC research. Fears of loss of prestige and prominence of local universities by the loss of investigators to California and the handful of other states where ESC research money is available is a powerful local political issue. The fact that Proposition 71 carried California by such a strong margin (59 percent), running ahead of Sen. Kerry, who easily carried the state, and gaining a majority in many conservative-leaning counties, indicated that the polls were correct; ESC research does resonate with voters.[11]

Although a year went by without further legislative action after the passage of HR 810, Senate action on a package of stem cell–related legislation, including HR 810, appears likely in the summer of 2006.[12] The bills to be considered in addition to HR 810 are not controversial and would promote research on non-embryo-derived alternative means to develop pluripotent cells and prohibit "embryo farming." It seems unlikely at this time that President Bush will change his approach or that HR 810, even if it should pass the Senate, will have enough support to override a veto. The president proposed additional restrictions in his 2005 State of the Union address: "I will work with Congress to ensure that human embryos are not created for experimentation or grown for body parts and that human life is never bought or sold as a commodity."

The president reiterated concerns about the direction of stem cell research in his 2006 State of the Union address when he said, "A hopeful society has institutions of science and medicine that do not cut ethical corners, and that recognize the matchless value of every life. Tonight I ask you to pass legislation to prohibit the most egregious abuses of medical research: human cloning in all its forms, creating or implanting embryos for experiments, creating human-animal hybrids, and buying, selling, or patenting human embryos. Human life is a gift from our Creator—and that gift should never be discarded, devalued or put up for sale."[13] However, no follow-up legislation was proposed after either speech, and the passage of HR 810 indicates that any legislative attempt to significantly restrict ESC research is now unlikely to succeed. The year 2006 may yet see a major test of resolve on both sides as federal legislation comes to its final phases.

ANTICLONING LEGISLATION

No issue illustrates the principle that is the title of this essay more than the issue of reproductive cloning. Interest in prohibiting reproductive cloning as a policy issue came to the fore shortly after the successful cloning of the sheep known as "Dolly."

Human reproductive cloning has been denounced by virtually all who have considered it. The National Research Council declared it to be "dangerous and likely to fail" and urged its prohibition.[14] Since the opposition to cloning is widespread and the only support for reproductive cloning is scattered and eccentric, one would expect that it would be quite straightforward to legislate a reasoned prohibition of human reproductive cloning. In fact, it has been difficult and contentious because the procedures of nuclear transfer that are central to cloning could also be used for the generation of blastocysts, and subsequently ESCs, for research and possibly therapeutic purposes. Thus the debate has been how to manage human nuclear transfer technology (or "therapeutic cloning") while outlawing reproductive cloning.

There have been two competing legislative strategies on this issue, with one approach attempting to regulate the technology and the other dealing with the outcome. These competing strategies allow little room for compromise and have resulted in failures to accomplish anything substantial either in the United States or at the United Nations. The first approach is exemplified by HR 1357, the Human Cloning Prohibition Act of 2005, proposed by Representatives Weldon (R-FL) and Stupak

(D-MI).[15] This legislation would amend the federal criminal code "to prohibit any person or entity, in or affecting interstate commerce, from knowingly: (1) performing or attempting to perform human cloning; (2) participating in such an attempt; (3) shipping or receiving an embryo produced by human cloning or any product derived from such embryo; or (4) importing such an embryo or derived product." Penalties of up to ten years in prison and fines up to $1 million are set forth. This legislation is quite a radical and unprecedented departure for American science policy in that it criminalizes not only an overt antisocial act but also an entire avenue of biomedical research. This approach ignores the traditional avenue of creating policy by determining if the federal government wishes to invest its resources in that area of research. (Representative Weldon has also tried that approach, seeking unsuccessfully in June 2005 to amend the NIH appropriation to prohibit the use of NIH funds for cloning research.)

One major problem with a comprehensive cloning ban that included nuclear transfer technology would be the very difficult enforcement issues. For example, would a patient who went to another country to receive therapy with stem cells derived by somatic cell nuclear transfer be subject to arrest upon return for importation of a banned material? Would an assisted reproduction specialist really be arrested for performing noncloning somatic transfer in order to avoid the certain inheritance of mitochondrial disease–associated mutations? How would our society react to the imprisonment of a scientist for studying breast cancer by generating an embryonic stem cell line with an inherited mutation of a gene such as BrCa1? But these questions have not been the central part of the political argument; the potential of these materials, however miniscule, to result in a human life is the sole focus of this legislation. Although HR 1137 has not been considered in 2005 or 2006, similar legislation easily passed the House in 2002 and 2003 and enjoyed the endorsement of President Bush. The comparable bill in the Senate (S 658) has never come to a vote, so its fate in that chamber is uncertain.

The alternative approach has been championed by a bipartisan coalition in the form of S 876. This proposed legislation would prohibit the act of attempting to actually produce a cloned human being, and it sets out a series of ethical guidelines for performing research using somatic cell nuclear transfer. This act has also not come to a vote, as any legislation in this contentious area would need sixty votes to overcome a filibuster. The Senate seems, at present, at an impasse. The failure to produce anticloning laws should not suggest that reproductive cloning could be done without restriction in the United States. In 1997 President Clinton issued a presidential directive prohibiting the use of federal funding for such research, once again emphasizing the tradition of using the power of federal support to mold science policy.[16] Even more potent was the assertion shortly thereafter of regulatory control over human reproductive cloning by the Food and Drug Administration.[17] This control should be adequate to root out any rogue laboratories that might think of this country as a safe haven for generating cloned humans.

The same contrasting approaches characterized the last several years of debate on cloning at the United Nations.[18] An initial resolution in 2001 by France and Germany launched an effort to develop a treaty banning reproductive cloning along with a second effort to arrive at a consensus on the ethical boundaries for research. However, the United States vigorously opposed a two-step approach and backed a resolution by Costa Rica that would have banned all forms of human cloning, including laboratory research. A competing resolution sponsored by South Korea and Belgium, and endorsed by national academies of science in more than sixty nations, returned to the original concept of banning only reproductive cloning. Since neither resolution had overwhelming support, a bloc of Islamic nations proposed a two-year postponement. The postponement passed, 80–79. This year the treaty approach was abandoned and a vaguely worded nonbinding advisory resolution opposing all forms of cloning passed 84–34 with thirty-seven abstentions.

What was perceived as wrong with the simple approach of a treaty banning reproductive cloning? After all, nearly everyone agrees that this would be a dangerous way to perpetuate our species. Apparently many delegations, including prominently the United States, felt that any failure to limit the use of cloning technology was the equivalent of endorsing the creation of embryos for research. Thus the opportunity was lost for worldwide agreement to establish a standard of scientific and medical behavior. We are unlikely to see a more acute example of the perfect as the lethal enemy of the good, as demanding a prohibition on all types of cloning, including research, prevented an agreement that might actually have had some impact on world opinion and might have had the salutary effect of establishing a world standard. Unfortunately, this opportunity is probably lost for the foreseeable future.

STATES AND ESC RESEARCH

The very limited federal support available for the rapidly developing field of ESC research left a vacuum, and several of the states rushed in to fill the void. The leader in this charge is California, and the passage of Proposition 71 in November 2004, with its commitment of $3 billion in research funds over the next ten years, is now the standard against which other states must compete. The form of the support, the California Institute for Regenerative Medicine (CIRM), is also a model for how such support can be structured, and it is an important precedent in government investment in biomedical science.[19] CIRM is structured as an independent agency with an already committed budget. In contrast to NIH, the National Science Foundation, and nearly all other science agencies, CIRM does not have to go back to the legislature annually for its appropriation. CIRM is governed by an Independent Citizens Oversight Committee (ICOC), which is dominated by representatives of patient advocates and academics, the alliance that so effectively campaigned for the passage of Proposition 71. The handing of this large responsibility to an agency outside the immediate reach of the legislature has bothered some legislators and is the subject of considerable legislative and legal wrangling. In fact, court challenges to Proposition 71 have delayed its full implementation well into 2006 and perhaps even later. Nonetheless, it is the model being considered in other states. For example, New York is considering legislation to support ESC research that would create a structure almost identical to CIRM.[20] One New York assemblyman, a co-sponsor of this legislation, told me that he believes support of medical research is a federal responsibility and that the state of New York should not have to use its resources there. But the absence of federal support and the specter of other states scooping up the best talent from New York universities and biotechnology companies was unacceptable, so he felt compelled to propose state support for ESC research.

In addition to California, several other states have moved forward to guarantee the legality of ESC research and provide funding for it.[21] New Jersey was the first, enacting legislation to protect ESC research in 2002. Following California's legislation and passage of Prop 71, Connecticut, Massachusetts, and Maryland passed enabling legislation to move into this field. New Jersey, Wisconsin, Illinois, Connecticut, and Maryland joined California in devoting state funding to this area of research. Massachusetts previously had a conflicting and confusing legal framework, and the 2005 legislation created a clear set of guidelines for research in this area. It passed over the veto of Governor Romney, who urged the deletion of protection for research using nuclear transfer. ESC permissive or supportive legislation is pending in several other states as well.

On the other side, more states have laws that restrict research with fetal or embryonic tissues, although only a few specifically mention embryonic stem cells. Currently, sixteen states have laws that specifically prohibit research on a human fetus or embryo, although the variety of definitions used for the materials that are excluded makes the situation difficult to summarize. For example, California, with its very permissive structure, also has existing law that prohibits the research use of aborted live fetuses. Most of the prohibitions appear to be aimed at prohibiting or severely limiting the use of aborted fetuses for research. Ten states have consent provisions that govern the use of aborted or fetal materials, and three (California, Connecticut, Massachusetts) have consent provisions that specifically govern the donation for research of materials from IVF procedures.

Seventeen states, mostly in the Midwest and the South, have laws that prohibit the use of fetal or embryonic materials obtained by means other than abortions. Most relevantly, six states (Arkansas, Indiana, Iowa, Michigan, North Dakota, and Virginia) have language that specifically prohibits research using human cloned embryos, and Louisiana specifically prohibits any research on embryos obtained from IVF procedures. Several states (Missouri, Nebraska, and Arizona) have reverted to the old model of limiting prohibitions to those actions that use state funds. For the rest of the states, what is illegal is illegal no matter what the funding source. President Bush's concern about the commercial sale of embryos has been addressed by half the states, as twenty-five states already have laws on the books that restrict or prohibit the sale of embryonic or fetal materials. Twenty states have not enacted any legislation that directly speaks to stem cell research, cloning, or related issues.

In summary, the individual states have moved ahead along the exact same dividing lines as the nation. Several states where biotechnology and research universities are central to the state image and economic strategy have moved decisively to protect ESC research and to promote it. Other state legislatures see the protection of embryos or fetuses as the central issue and have passed legislation that restricts or prohibits ESC research. Most of the action thus far has been within state legislatures, and it will be interesting to see if popular referenda will be tried in other states besides California. Missouri will also be the next test of the appeal of stem cells at the ballot box as it votes in 2006 on a referendum that would preclude any restrictions on research that are more stringent than federal law.

CONCLUSIONS

ESC research has proven to be an almost insurmountable challenge for science policy makers. Compromise is not easy to reach, as there are no examples of working compromises that both ESC advocates and opponents can live with and publicly support. Given that fact, it is not surprising that both sides move ahead wherever they can, with ESC proponents building support in states on the West Coast, the Northeast, and the Great Lakes area, while state legislatures in the South, the Midwest, and Plains states are busy making the same research illegal. This situation is not entirely unprecedented, since science issues as diverse as environmental protection and the teaching of evolution have long divided the various states. However, with Congress moving slowly on stem cell legislation and with a president not inclined to change the current policy, we are unlikely to establish a national standard that will guide the individual states. Thus we are likely to see more, not less, action at the state level on the ESC issue.

If the perfect is the enemy of the good, have we lost good things in this debate as each side searched for perfect outcomes? I fear that we have. The first loss is the almost complete erosion of the compromise that governed research on embryonic materials: the restriction of federal research support to embryonic materials already obtained with nonfederal funds. This compromise seems irretrievable now. The second loss is the loss of the ability to have a national consensus on an issue of great scientific importance, resulting in a patchwork of state policies that will only serve to further concentrate biomedical research in a relatively small cluster of states. Finally, we will have lost time in testing and developing this exciting area of research. That loss is irreplaceable.

NOTES

1. Withdrawal of interim NIH guidelines for the support and conduct of therapeutic human fetal tissue transplantation research in light of superseding provisions of Public Law 103–43, the National Institutes of Health Revitalization Act of 1993. See *NIH Guide* 22 (Sept. 3, 1993).

2. Kyla Dunn, "The Politics of Stem Cells," *Nova Science Now*, April 15, 2005, www.pbs.org/wgbh/nova/sciencenow/dispatches/050413.html (accessed Jan. 8, 2007).

3. "President Discusses Stem Cell Research," White House news release, Aug. 9, 2001, www.whitehouse.gov/news/releases/2001/08/20010809-2.html (accessed Jan. 8, 2007).

4. Jocelyn Kaiser, "Interview: Elias Zerhouni: Taking Stock," *Science* 308 (June 3, 2005): 1398–99.

5. "Letter from FASEB President Robert Rich to President Bush," Aug. 31, 2001, http://opa.faseb.org/pdf/stem8.31.01.pdf (accessed Jan. 8, 2007).

6. "Why Federal Stem Cell Policy Must Be Expanded," JDRF Scientific White Paper, August 2004, www.jdrf.org/files/About_JDRF/JDRF%20Stem%20Cell%20White%20Paper%202004.pdf (accessed February 9, 2007).

7. David Malakoff, "Election 2004: The Calculus of Making Stem Cells a Campaign Issue," *Science* 305 (Aug. 6, 2004): 760.

8. Senator Sam Brownback, "Embryonic Stem Cell Research," http://brownback.senate.gov/LIStemCell.cfm (accessed Jan. 8, 2007).

9. Stephen S. Hall, *Merchants of Immortality* (Boston: Houghton Mifflin, 2003), 272–76.

10. "H.R. 810," THOMAS (Library of Congress) Web site, http://thomas.loc.gov/cgi-bin/bdquery/z?d109:h.r.00810:. (accessed Jan. 8, 2007).

11. California Secretary of State, "Vote 2004," www.ss.ca.gov/elections/sov/2004_general/contents.htm (accessed Jan. 8, 2007).

12. Constance Holden, "Senate Prepares to Vote at Last on a Trio of Stem Cell Bills," *Science* 313 (July 7, 2006): 27–28.

13. George W. Bush, State of the Union Address, 2005, www.whitehouse.gov/state of the union/2005/index.html, and State of the Union Address, 2006, www.whitehouse.gov/stateoftheunion/2006/index.html (accessed Jan. 8, 2007).

14. Committee on Science, Engineering, and Public Policy and Board of Life Sciences, *Scientific and Medical Aspects of Human Reproductive Cloning* (Washington, DC: National Research Council, 2002), available online at www.nap.edu/books/0309076374/html/.

15. "H.R. 1357," THOMAS (Library of Congress) Web site, http://thomas.loc.gov/cgi-bin/bdquerytr/z?d109:HR01357: (accessed Jan. 8, 2007).

16. President William J. Clinton, "Presidential Directive: Prohibition on Federal Funding for Cloning of Human Beings," March 4, 1997, http://grants.nih.gov/grants/policy/cloning_directive.htm (accessed Jan. 8, 2007).

17. U.S. Food and Drug Administration, "Use of Cloning Technology to Clone a Human Being," Dec. 27, 2002, www.fda.gov/cber/genetherapy/clone.htm (accessed Jan. 8, 2007).

18. Center for Genetics and Society, "Human Cloning, the United Nations, and Beyond," 2003, modified April 15, 2004, www.genetics-and-society.org/policies/international/2003unreport.html (accessed Jan. 8, 2007).

19. See the Web site of the California Institute for Regenerative Medicine, www.cirm.ca.gov/.

20. "New York State Assembly Bill Number 06300," http://assembly.state.ny.us/leg/?bn = 6300 (accessed Jan. 8, 2007).

21. National Conference of State Legislatures, "State Embryonic and Fetal Research Laws," updated Dec. 5, 2006, www.ncsl.org/programs/health/genetics/embfet.htm (accessed Jan. 8, 2007).

CHAPTER 8

Ethical Issues in Stem Cell Research, Therapy, and Public Policy

Ronald B. Miller

Stem cell research, therapy, and public policy engender issues that are heatedly debated and variably regulated in the United States. Today's ethical issues are likely to determine tomorrow's public policy (legislation and regulation) even if widespread consensus is not achieved. Let me begin, then, by defining how I will use the terms *ethics* and *morality*, even though later in the discussion we may find it enlightening to understand the terms as defined differently by Stanford philosopher Ernle W. D. Young. The adjectives *ethical* and *moral* are commonly used as if they were synonymous, but the nouns are not. Although neither *ethics* nor *morality* is uniformly defined, I find it useful to define *morality* as a tradition (whether religious, cultural, or professional) of what is good, right, and just (or bad, wrong, and unjust) and *ethics* as a discipline of either theology or philosophy that studies morality—that is, studies religious, cultural, and professional views of what is good, right, and just.

Of necessity the law is pragmatically minimalist whereas ethics is aspirational or maximalist. Legislative law codifies, and case law reaffirms, the ethical principles, beliefs, or judgments that have achieved sufficient public consensus to be adopted or enforced. Regulations, however, are often adopted before there is public consensus. Some of what I will address has achieved consensus, but some is gestating and is often debated rather than discussed.

I will begin with a brief review of normal embryologic development and of the sources of stem cells, a statement of ethical goals for stem cell research, and a review of two matters of general societal agreement and two matters of major societal disagreement that complicate—if not prevent—the development of satisfactory, coherent public policy. I will then review religious as well as secular ethical beliefs and concepts fundamental to a subsequent overview of the ethical issues for stem cell research, for stem cell therapy, and for stem cell policy development. I will conclude with selected opinions regarding whether we can achieve societal consensus and possible approaches to doing so, as well as my personal opinions regarding stem cell research.

A BRIEF REVIEW OF NORMAL HUMAN EMBRYOLOGIC DEVELOPMENT

This review or overview is provided to facilitate understanding of the ethical and policy issues in stem cell research and therapy. I have chosen to employ the term *pre-embryo* for the first two weeks of human development (rather than considering that the embryo begins at the time of syngamy or fertilization) because it provides a logical basis for assigning greater moral status as development progresses. However, as the renowned Catholic theologian Richard A. McCormick, S.J., of the University of Notre Dame (who was a member of the federal Ethics Advisory Board and the Ethics Committee of the American Fertility Society) pointed out, the term was adopted by the American Fertility Society not "as an exercise of linguistic engineering to make human embryo research more palatable to the general public" (Jarmulowicz 1990, 181) but "because the earliest stages of mammalian development primarily involve establishment of the non-embryonic trophoblast, rather than the formation of the embryo" (McCormick 1991, 1). "The scientific rationale for the term 'pre-embryo' . . . is its greater accuracy in characterizing the initial phase of mammalian development" (Grobstein 1988, 61). Lest one believe the term *pre-embryo* outdated, Carson Strong, in a 2005 article in the *American Journal of Bioethics*, stated, "It is accepted practice in the bioethics literature to refer to the human conceptus prior to the formation of the primitive streak . . . as the 'pre-embryo' " (21). For a more detailed and sophisticated understanding of human embryologic development, the reader is referred to chapter 1 of this book, by Peter Bryant, and chapter 2, by Philip Schwartz and Peter Bryant.

A *gamete* is an oocyte (egg) or a spermatozoon (sperm). Each contains half the number of chromosomes of all other cells of the body. A *zygote* is a fertilized egg, the result of the union of egg and sperm. It is totipotent—that is, able to form all cell types, including those of the chorionic portion of the placenta as well as of the fetus, and thus in utero it has the capacity to develop into an organism. It cleaves (divides) repeatedly over three to four days without any overall growth in size (i.e., the cells double in number but become smaller). Up to at least the eight-cell stage, each cell is totipotent and could become an entire organism if separated from the others. As it divides further, it becomes a *morula,* a solid mass of sixteen to thirty-two cells that looks like a mulberry. Each of its cells is called a *blastomere,* and with successive cell divisions the cells become smaller though the size of the morula remains the same.

The mass of cells begins to hollow out, and at four to seven days after fertilization and seven or eight sets of cell division it becomes a *blastocyst* (which is 0.1–0.2 mm in diameter, about the size of the dot of an i or a period on this page). The blastocyst (also called a blastula) is a hollow sphere of 50 to 250 cells (surrounding a fluid-filled cavity, the blastocoel), many of which cells (the outer layer or *trophoblast*), if implanted in the uterus, would become the chorion (the embryonic portion of the *placenta*) but twenty to thirty of which are the inner cell mass that would become the embryo (and the yolk sac, the allantois, and the amnion) and later the fetus. The *yolk sac* (for nutrition in birds and reptiles but not mammals) manufactures early blood cells and germ cells. The *allantois* is the waste sac prior to placental function and kidney development, and the *amnion* is the water sac, which serves as an intrauterine shock absorber for the fetus (Gilbert et al. 2005). The blastocyst implants in the uterus five to eight days following conception. The chorion secretes a hormone (human chorionic gonadotrophin) that induces the ovary to secrete progesterone, which causes the uterus to remain soft and malleable (and enlarge as the fetus grows). The chorion also produces chemicals that block the maternal immune system so that the embryo and fetus will not be miscarried (Gilbert at al. 2005). The embryonic blood vessels of the chorion come into contact with maternal blood vessels in the *decidua* (the maternal portion of the placenta), allowing nutrition from, and waste excretion to, the mother.

With further cell divisions over another week and further invagination of cells, the blastula becomes the *gastrula.* The invagination of cells begins on about day 14 and forms the three primary germ layers of the gastrula: (1) *ectoderm,* which will become skin, nervous tissue, eyes, ears, and breasts; (2) *mesoderm,* which will become blood cells and vessels, heart, spleen and lymphatics, kidneys, gonads, connective tissue, bone, muscle, and fat; and (3) *endoderm,* which will become lungs, liver, pancreas, gut, bladder, tonsils, pharynx, and parathyroid glands.

The gastrula at fourteen days has approximately two thousand cells and begins to develop the *primitive streak,* the first marker or anlage of the nervous system. Prior to this, the pre-embryo can feel no pain since it has no nervous system. (Indeed, it is not until approximately the twenty-third week that the fetus can respond to painful stimuli [Craig et al. 1993].) Furthermore, prior to this developmental milestone at twelve to fourteen days, the pre-embryo could divide to form twins, and in this sense individuality (which is essential in the minds of many to identity and personhood) has not yet been established. Thus scientists and ethicists have proposed that research on the developing organism should be limited to the first fourteen days after conception (Ethics Advisory Board 1979).

From about two weeks to the seventh or eighth week, as the long axis of the body appears, the organism is called an *embryo.* It should be noted, however, that many apply the term *embryo* to the earlier developmental stages following conception as well as to the postimplantation phase of caudal-rostral (head-tail) differentiation. At one month the embryo is 3 mm long (the size of a pea).

When all the major structures (organs) have become evident at about seven to eight weeks, the embryo becomes a *fetus* for the remainder of the pregnancy and gestation (i.e., until birth). The fetus has all structures, organs, and a human form with recognizable limbs, brain, eyes, ears, nose, heart, and a nervous system. After two months, development is primarily growth and maturation. At twenty-three to twenty-five weeks the fetus is viable and might be called a *vionate,* and at thirty-eight to forty weeks it is born a full-term *neonate.*

STEM CELLS AND THEIR SOURCES

As previously noted, as the zygote (the fertilized egg) divides, at least up to the eight-cell stage, the cells are thought to be *totipotent:* that is, each cell could become an entire organism as well as the chorionic portion of the placenta and could become any cell of the entire body, which has more than two hundred cell types. Pre-embryonic or blastocystic stem cells (usually called *embryonic stem cells*) are *pluripotent,* as are fetal germ cells from the gonadal ridge and as perhaps are amniotic fluid (De-Coppi et al. 2007), umbilical cord, and placental stem cells.[1] That is, they can become any cell of the entire organism excluding the chorion (i.e., any cell of the body). Experimentally *pre-embryonic or blastocystic stem cells* are obtained in the laboratory from the inner cell mass of a blastocyst that has not been placed in the uterus for implantation—that is, they are *preimplantation stem cells*. Theoretically at least, the cells of the implanted blastocyst or early embryo would also be pluripotent.

Embryonic or fetal germ cells are also pluripotent (Gearhart 1998; Shamblott et al. 1998), though possibly slightly less so than blastocystic stem cells. Embryonic or fetal germ cells are obtained from the gonadal ridge (what will become ovarian or testicular tissue) of a spontaneously or electively aborted embryo or fetus five to nine weeks after conception.

Umbilical cord and placental stem cells are also thought to be pluripotent, though possibly less so than earlier stem cells. Stem cells can be obtained from amniotic fluid (DeCoppi et al. 2007), from the blood of the umbilical cord, and in even greater numbers from Wharton's jelly (Wang et al. 2004), the connective tissue of the umbilical cord. Like Wharton's jelly, the placenta is a rich source of stem cells (Fukuchi et al. 2004).

Stem cells are capable of both symmetric division (self-renewal or the production of two undifferentiated cells) and asymmetric division (producing one undifferentiated and one at least partially differentiated cell). A *stem cell line* is the undifferentiated progeny of a stem cell—that is, the mass of stem cells that are produced in vitro by repeated symmetric cell divisions without differentiation into specialized cell types or tissues. *Nonembryonic* stem cells, also called *mature* stem cells or *adult* stem cells, are undifferentiated cells in a differentiated tissue, and they have somewhat less "potency": often they are multipotent rather than pluripotent. The anatomic location in which adult stem cells reside is called a niche. Presumably these cells are responsible for the normal repair of tissues and organs that are damaged by disease or senescence. The niche may somehow determine or regulate how stem cells are sustained and how they participate in tissue repair (Scadden 2006). Quite possibly this is achieved through growth or paracrine factors (chemicals that bind to receptors and alter cell activity but that, unlike hormones that circulate in the blood, are located in the tissue they affect [Gilbert et al. 2005]). As well as being less potent, adult stem cells do not have the same ability as embryonic stem cells to divide indefinitely and to grow large numbers of cells in vitro. Adult stem cells are less flexible or plastic (less able to transdifferentiate into cells of a different tissue than that of the tissue from which they came) than embryonic stem cells (at least to date—though one hopes we will learn how to dedifferentiate such cells such that when they are again differentiated they can become many, if not all, cell types). Examples of so-called adult stem cells are the hematopoietic stem cells of the bone marrow (which can form red blood cells, white blood cells—including those of the immune system—and platelets), and neural stem cells, which can form the three major types of cells in the brain (neurons, astrocytes, and oligodendrocytes). It has been reported (National Research Council/Institute of Medicine 2002) that both hematopoietic and neural stem cells are plastic: that is, each can give rise to the differentiated cells of the other! However, Irving Weissman (pers. comm., March 9, 2007) believes that this transdifferentiation has not been proven. Other lineage-specific stem cells include skin, hair follicle, dental, cardiac and skeletal muscle, and male (but not female) germinal stem cells (Gilbert et al. 2005). *Progenitor* or *precursor cells* are early descendents of stem cells that have limited ability to differentiate (less potency) but no ability to self-renew; the lack of asymmetric cell division distinguishes them from stem cells. Stem cells were identified in 1981 in mice (Evans and Kaufman 1981; Martin 1981) and were first isolated in 1988 from human blastocysts (Thomson et al. 1998) and from human fetal germ cells (Gearhart 1988), though hematopoietic stem cells (before they were known as stem cells) had been transplanted as bone marrow (after radiation or chemotherapeutic destruction of a patient's own leukemic bone marrow) since the 1960s. It is now believed that there are leukemia stem cells and cancer stem cells and that if these "are isolated and transplanted into immunodeficient mice, such tumor-bearing mice should be useful for preclinical testing of diagnostics and drug and immune therapy" (Weissman 2005, 1363). For those who wish a more detailed and illustrated review of stem cells, I recommend a booklet that can be downloaded from www.nationalacademies.org/stem cells (National Academies 2007b).

GOALS OF STEM CELL RESEARCH

James Childress of the University of Virginia defined the goals of stem cell research as follows: while respecting the dignity of stem cells that are nascent human life, to realize the therapeutic promise of stem cells to alleviate human suffering (pursuing all avenues of research to this end) and thereafter to make stem cell therapy available equitably (Childress 2004). And as Lori Knowles of the Hasting Center wrote in a commissioned paper (for the National Bioethics Advisory Commission, chaired by the then-president of Princeton, Harold Shapiro), stem cell research requires respect for human life and dignity; quality and safety of research and treatment; free, informed consent for each; and goals of relief of human suffering, freedom of research investigation, wide availability of the knowledge that is generated, and noncommercialization of reproduction and donation (Knowles 2000, H-6; National Bioethics Advisory Commission 2000, H-6). To these, I would add research integrity and avoidance of complicity in inappropriate research by either the subject or the investigator. The goals and requirements noted by Knowles are expressed in terms that warrant virtually universal acceptance, since they apply to research with mature, nonembryonic, adult stem cells as well as to research with embryonic stem cells.

TWO COMMON SOCIETAL AGREEMENTS

There is general societal consensus in the United States regarding two fundamental conceptions of stem cells and of stem cell research. Together, however, they form the crux of an ethical dilemma, as they are in tension with each other.

1. The blastocyst (which currently must be destroyed to obtain/harvest the inner cells that are stem cells) is human, and thus deserving of respect, and must not be treated with wanton disregard. Some would emphasize that although it is human it is not a human being or person. Even so, we have a duty to respect it, even if not always to protect it, since—given a supportive environment and good luck (or God's grace)—it has the potential to become a child.

2. The potential of stem cell research to result in remarkable therapies is an expectant boon to mankind. Stem cell research should yield at least seven benefits:

    a. An understanding of normal and abnormal development (cellular differentiation and function);

    b. An understanding of disease mechanisms such as the uninhibited growth of cancer cells; and thus

    c. Amelioration or cure of diseases;

    d. The design of effective therapy with drugs targeted at basic mechanisms, established by research with cells in vitro rather than with animals or humans;

    e. The repair or replacement of degenerated, damaged, or destroyed tissues or organs—for example, return of spinal cord function following injury by injection of stem cells that minimize scarring and stimulate the release of growth factors that effect repair (thus far these appear to be the primary mechanisms in animals injected with stem cells—after experimental spinal cord injury—that might have been thought to grow new neurons);

f. Ability to grow organs in vitro and/or in vivo to lessen dependence on cadaveric and live-donor organs for transplantation, since organs are in such short supply that recipients often wait two to five years for a transplant (and many unfortunately die waiting); and

g. Hopefully avoiding immunologic rejection, which at least currently requires somatic cell nuclear transfer (SCNT) from the patient (who is the potential tissue or organ recipient) to a donor egg whose nucleus has been removed. Another fascinating approach that was hoped might achieve true immune tolerance is the creation of a mixed chimera, a technique called co-transplantation. The experimental animal or human to receive a kidney transplant is also given sublethal irradiation or chemotherapy to markedly reduce but not permanently eradicate the individual's immune system and is then infused with hematopoietic stem cells of the same donor as the kidney. Although this has not produced complete tolerance, markedly less immunosuppression is required (Millan et al. 2002; Strober et al. 2004).

Because of these likely potential benefits, many believe that scientists and physicians have a duty to conduct stem cell research and that the moral issues have been thoroughly considered (Moreno and Berger 2006), but for some scientists this duty conflicts with a conscientiously held duty to not only respect but protect the blastocyst, the pre-embryonic source of stem cells. Similarly ethical objections to therapeutic cloning (SCNT) and to oocyte donation for the purpose of research may preclude the use of embryonic stem cells.

TWO MAJOR SOCIETAL DISAGREEMENTS

The first (and fundamental) disagreement is the degree of regard for or respect due to the blastocyst (the pre-embryo) and whether it can be sacrificed for research or for the therapeutic benefit of other humans. As noted, the blastocyst (the five-day pre-embryo) has no nervous system (and therefore no feeling), no human form, no brain (and thus no awareness of pain even if it had feeling), no heart, no lungs, no stomach, no kidneys, not even legs to run away. The twenty to thirty cells of the inner cell mass can be isolated (removed from the blastocyst) and grown separately in vitro in the laboratory for research or for therapy. The inner cells are pluripotent embryonic stem cells. An interesting notion regarding the moral status of the blastocyst is based upon its lack of even a neural crest—that is, its total lack of a brain or nervous system. Jeffrey Kahn (Kahn 2004) and Michael Gazzaniga (2005, 8) point out that at the other extreme of life, when an individual's brain dies, we pronounce death by neurologic criteria and can transplant organs, perform a postmortem examination, and bury the corpse. Why not the same with the blastocyst, which has no brain? An obvious possible answer: because it has the potential to develop a brain.

The second disagreement: some believe the controversy could be avoided entirely by using nonembryonic stem cells (so-called adult stem cells). Unfortunately, they are more difficult to isolate and more difficult to grow: they have a lesser ability to self-replicate, and some replicate more slowly and only a limited number of times. This is true of embryonic germ cells as well. Furthermore, some organs appear not to have adult stem cells (Gilbert et al. 2005). And even if we learn how to grow them in large numbers and how to stimulate them to become multiple different cell or tissue types (which may require a degree of dedifferentiation before stimulating them to differentiate to the desired cell type), if they are not autologous there is still the problem of immunologic rejection, just as there is from transplantation of organs other than between identical twins. A potential solution to this problem of rejection of foreign stem cells is SCNT (commonly called therapeutic cloning), in which the nucleus of a somatic cell (e.g., a skin cell) from the specific patient who needs the stem cell therapy is placed into a donated enucleated oocyte (egg) and stimulated to divide and become a blastocyst. The stem cells (i.e., the inner cell mass of that blastocyst), then, have nearly the identical genetic makeup (differing only in the mitochondrial DNA of the enucleated egg) of the patient needing the stem cell therapy, so that immunologic rejection is much less likely than when stem cells obtained from in vitro fertilization (IVF)-discarded embryos (which have different nuclear DNA from that of the recipient) are implanted or infused into the patient. Although many have ignored the mitochondria of the enucleated egg in SCNT, and although it may be much less of a problem when the somatic cell nucleus and the enucleated egg are from two individuals of the same species (Cascalnho and Platt 2005; Lanza et al. 2002), Douglas Wallace of the University of California, Irvine warns that the problem may be vastly greater if the egg is of a different species from that of the somatic cell (Dennis 2006).

Even though therapeutic cloning begins with (and employs the DNA of) a differentiated somatic cell rather than with a fertilized oocyte, since it proceeds to cell multiplication (after implantation in an enucleated oocyte) and the formation of a blastocyst (which, if implanted in a uterus, could become a fetus), the sacrifice of that blastocyst to obtain stem cells is thought ethically impermissible by those who believe that a blastocyst that results from growth of an egg fertilized in vitro (a zygote) must not be sacrificed (even though reproductive "cloning" is not involved). Yet another concern or fear is expressed in the "slippery slope" argument that therapeutic cloning would lead to reproductive cloning (i.e., concern that a cloned blastocyst would be allowed to develop into a human child). Because of risks of physical abnormalities and because of psychological burdens for such a child, even if reproductive cloning were technically possible (which Hyun and Jung 2006 state it is not because of the fragility of primate eggs), it is currently considered unethical and is uniformly opposed by the same scientific and medical communities that overwhelmingly support stem cell research with both embryonic (whether from "spare" IVF embryos or from SCNT) and adult stem cells. Not all agree it is an equivalent concern: Paul McHugh (2004) of the President's Council on Bioethics argues that a "clonote" (the product of SCNT) is "a product of biologic manufacturing, and may therefore ethically be used to derive embryonic stem cells." However, those who object to the word *pre-embryo* may similarly object to the term *clonote,* believing that these words call the organism by a different name simply to diminish its ethical status.

"In scientific parlance, cloning is a broadly used, shorthand term that refers to producing a copy of some biological entity—a gene, an organism, a cell" (Vogelstein et al. 2002, 1237). As the authors note, "Much confusion has arisen in the public, in that cloning seems to have become almost synonymous with somatic cell nuclear transfer, a procedure that can be used for many different purposes. Only one of these purposes involves an intention to create a clone of the organism (for example, a human)." Two other extremely important potential uses of SCNT are (1) to create stem cells genetically identical to a patient who needs replacement of a tissue or organ (thereby avoiding immune rejection) and (2) to create stem cell lines from the somatic cells of a patient with a genetic disorder that would allow study of the nature and possible treatment of the disorder. The latter two uses have led to the popular term *therapeutic cloning* (which is easily confused with *reproductive cloning*) to distinguish these two purposes from the first without resorting to the more difficult term *somatic cell nuclear transfer*. And this leads to even further confusion, since some speak of reproductive cloning as "therapeutic" for infertility. Thus the authors have titled their article "Please Don't Call It Cloning!" and they recommend the term *nuclear transplantation*. Whether we call it *nuclear transplantation* or *nuclear transfer*, I agree we should eliminate *therapeutic cloning* from our lexicon.

SECULAR AND RELIGIOUS ETHICAL TENETS

The central controversy about the degree of regard or moral respect due the blastocyst, and thus its rights, can be discussed as the *moral status* or *moral worth* of the blastocyst. Alternatively, as suggested by the President's Council on Bioethics, the moral status is epitomized by the question "When does life begin?" (President's Council on Bioethics 2003; 2004b, 74). Although all agree the blastocyst is human and is living, some hold this mass of thirty cells that is barely visible and only the size of the point of a pin (0.1 or 0.2 mm in diameter) has no human form, has no nervous system, is not a person or a human being, and has no soul and thus need not be accorded the protection due persons, human beings, or ensouled beings.

Others, however, believe that from the very moment of conception, because the zygote-morula-blastocyst has the potential to become a child and eventually an adult, it has full moral status and must not be harmed or destroyed. From this perspective, to do so is to treat it as a means only and not as an end in itself, and to commit murder and violate God's will. This deontologic perspective is often an absolutist position, inflexible, and held with deep moral conviction.

In contrast, those who believe the blastocyst does not have full moral status hold an instrumental view or notion of moral status dependent upon the degree of development of the human organism. Ted Peters, following concepts of Daniel Callahan, distinguishes three basic ethical schools of thought (Geron Ethics Advisory Board 1999, 32):

1. Genetic determinism: life and moral status begin at conception

2. The developmental view: life begins at conception, but moral status depends upon the degree of development

3. The social view: personhood and moral status are social constructs

To these I would add a fourth:

4. The religious view: ensoulment is the basis of moral status, and various religions have different concepts of when it occurs. It is often thought to require a formed body, which marks the transition from embryo to fetus at approximately two months of gestation (Peterson 2003; Reichardt et al. 2004).

With regard to the developmentalist/incrementalist view of moral status (items 2 and 4 above), most agree that a human conceptus, no matter how young or undeveloped, has greater moral status than a gamete (egg or sperm), and greater status also than a subhuman animal or certainly than plant life. Only some of us would go on to say the blastocyst has greater value than a zygote or morula, which has not yet implanted in the uterus, but perhaps we could agree that its moral value is less than that of a gastrula, with its three germ layers, or that of a neurula, whose primitive nervous system has begun, or that of an embryo or fetus, which would in turn have less moral value than a vionate or neonate, and they in turn less than a born child, and certainly less than an adolescent capable of functioning independently.

These incremental or developmental milestones are commonly thought to be morally relevant except by those who insist that all human life from the time of conception is sacred and of equal value. Another incrementalist notion, advanced by the late John Fletcher, accords varying moral status depending upon the source of the stem cells and the intentions of the donor(s). Moral status increases with each of the following:

Fetal tissue from a miscarriage (spontaneous abortion)

Cryogenically frozen embryos created in an IVF clinic but in excess of those needed by the couple (here I might add another level of distinction: those appearing abnormal and less likely to lead to successful pregnancy would have less moral status than those appearing healthy [Schwartz and Rae 2006])

Fetal tissue from an elective or "therapeutic" abortion

Embryos created by SCNT

Embryos created for the purpose of treating a sibling

Embryos created for the purpose of research (Fletcher 2000)

Yet another consideration is whether the moral status of the blastocyst depends in part upon its location: Is its moral status different if it is in vitro (in a petri dish or in a freezer in an IVF clinic) rather than in vivo (in the mother)? And is its moral status greater after implantation in the uterus than when the zygote is traveling down the fallopian tube? Note that loss of pre-embryos and embryos is "natural" (i.e., commonplace) in normal human reproduction, with perhaps as many as 80 percent of fertilized eggs failing to implant or of embryos miscarrying. And save for couples who have difficulty conceiving a child, this natural loss is not considered tragic (President's Council on Bioethics 2004b, 88).

Appreciate that there are at least three necessary conditions for the development of a human being or person: sperm, egg, and uterus (Guinin 2001, 2003), and to these I would add a fourth: a willing/consenting woman who allows her pregnancy to continue to viability. Mention of the gametes raises an interesting response to the question "When does life begin?" Are we really only interested in the question of when the life of an individual human begins? Are gametes not alive? Clearly they are important, but they are not the beginning of life, since they would be dead were they not in a live host. And that host would not be alive were it not for the gametes that formed her or him. This line of reasoning suggests that human life began when *Homo sapiens* evolved, and if one wishes not to restrict discussion of the beginning of life to our species, we again trace life through evolution; should we not say that it began with "the Big Bang"?

Personhood is an understandably popular secular notion related to moral status: that is, related to the degree of respect or value we ascribe to a developing human. There are problems, however, with the conventional criteria for personhood:

Consciousness: this criterion would include subhuman animals as
    persons.

Self-consciousness: this criterion would exclude normal infants.

Ability to reason: this criterion excludes the infant and also those
    with severe developmental delay or with dementia (Siegel 2000).

These views were considered by both the National Bioethics Advisory Commission (1999, regarding cloning) and the President's Council on Bioethics (2004b, regarding stem cells). The President's Council on Bioethics states that the issue ought to be understood either as (1) a matter of principle (respect for nascent human life, i.e, the inviolability of the human embryo or human life) or (2) a matter of balancing competing goods (the health benefits of stem cell research and the relief of suffering versus respect for nascent human life and protection of human life).

Bortolotti and Harris (2006) distinguish moral status (for which sentience is a necessary condition) from the moral value of nonsentient beings such as the pre-embryo (which value derives from symbolic significance). They prefer "to refrain from using arguments relying on symbolic value in the debate on stem cell research" (32) and from discussion of the moral status of the embryo. They believe that "symbolic value might track aesthetic preferences rather than morally relevant preferences" (33).

With regard to the notion of personhood and moral status, the "standard view" (the generally accepted commonsense view) of what makes it wrong to kill a person is that the person is human (Marquis 2006, 19, 21). Marquis, however, prefers a future-value account of moral status in which what makes it wrong to kill a person is that it deprives the person "of all of the goods of life that [he] otherwise would have experienced" (23). This "valuable future" or a "future-like-ours (FLO)" account is discussed in an accompanying article by Bonnie Steinbock (2006), who prefers to base "moral status on the possession of interests" that are protected by rights (human rights). She believes "the possession of interest is a necessary condition of having moral status, and . . . would argue that it is also a sufficient condition" (28). On the other hand, she argues that it is permissible to use embryos in research (so long as the research is not frivolous) because she believes that embryos lack moral status. Nevertheless, they should be treated respectfully because of their symbolic value, though this should not override the interests of sentient beings. And she states that if one accepts the future-value approach, it would be better to use SCNT embryos, since they lack an FLO, than to use embryos that might be discarded by an IVF clinic because they potentially have an FLO (Steinbock 2006).

It seems essential that we now consider views of the major religions that influence beliefs about the moral status of the conceptus (National Bioethics Advisory Commission 1999).[2] The current (since 1869 and Pope Pius IX) official position of the Roman Catholic Church is that ensoulment, personhood, and full moral status occur at conception (Reichardt et al. 2004). This has not always been the case, as Saint Thomas Aquinas (in views dating back to Aristotle) believed that ensoulment occurred at forty days after conception for boys, and at ninety days for girls. Catholic teaching is based upon notions of natural law and the duty to protect human life. IVF itself is seen as unnatural and wrong, and the use of excess IVF embryos is opposed because obtaining the stem cells destroys a human being: "the ablation of the inner cell mass (ICM) of the blastocyst, which critically and irremediably damages the human embryo, curtailing its development, is a gravely immoral act and consequently is gravely illicit" (Pontifical Academy for Life 2000, quoted in President's Council on Bioethics 2004b, 242). Catholicism, however, "does not oppose stem cell research per se" and—save for those who believe the use of aborted fetal tissue complicitly encourages abortion—permits, even encourages, the use of stem cells "from miscarried fetuses, placental [or cord] blood, and adult tissue" (National Bioethics Advisory Commission 1999, 99). Furthermore, some Catholics as well as the Eastern Orthodox Church support embryonic stem cell research utilizing cells from preexisting stem cell lines or from miscarriages (National Bioethics Advisory Commission 1999). Christianity has generally sanctioned animal research for the benefit of humans, though recent concern for their vulnerability and well-being dictates the minimization of harm to animal subjects (Gilbert et al. 2005).

Jewish principles hold that humans are only stewards of their bodies, which belong to God, and that humans "are God's partners in healing" (National Bioethics Advisory Commission 1999, 100). Because of *pikauch nefesh*, the duty to save a life and to heal, if stem cells have therapeutic promise, they should be employed (Scott 2006), and, as the President's Council stated, "Access to therapies developed through stem cell research is a crucial issue of justice for the Jewish community" (President's Council on Bioethics 2004b, 250).

In Conservative Judaism the fetus becomes a person at the fortieth day after the first missed menstrual period (and thus at approximately the fifty-sixth day after conception) but does not achieve full moral rights until birth (President's Council on Bioethics 2004b). Prior to the fortieth day the embryo (and by extension a frozen embryo in an IVF clinic) may be discarded or used for research (Gilbert et al. 2005). Further, in Conservative Judaism, abortion is obligatory if the mother's health is threatened, whereas in Orthodox Judaism the fetus develops full moral rights at the fortieth day, and abortion thereafter is homicide, though it is permissible to harvest stem cells from an abortus.

Judaism permits the experimental use of animals for the benefit of humans and especially human health but places more emphasis on animal welfare, avoidance of cruelty, and minimization of suffering than Christianity does (Gilbert et al. 2005). "Judaism and Christianity emphasize the unique dignity of human beings created in the image and likeness of God (imago Dei)" (Meyer 2000, 167).

Protestant views vary enormously, from prohibition of blastocyst destruction (Southern Baptist, Methodist, and Anglican) to permissibility justified by the benefit that may derive from stem cell research and therapy (Presbyterian and some Lutheran views). Respect is due the early embryo, but most Protestants believe there should be universal access to the benefits of research (Scott 2005; Gilbert et al. 2005).

In Islam personhood is a process, and personhood and ensoulment do not occur until the fourth month. Thus it is permissible to use embryos (whether created specifically for research or originally for IVF) to improve human health, and even illegitimately aborted fetuses may be used for good (National Bioethics Advisory Commission 1999; Gilbert et al. 2005). However, it is believed that "human disease is caused by humans and that animals need not suffer for this," and animal research is thought inappropriate (Gilbert et al. 2005).

Hindus believe in transmigration: at death the soul enters another body (animal or human) and flourishes or suffers depending on the individual's behavior or karma. However, transmigration is thought to be a predicament of endless cycles, and there is a quest to be liberated from the repeated cycles of birth and death and to enter a state of timeless bliss. Although all life is sacred, birth of a girl is thought unfortunate and may even occasion infanticide, although both infanticide and abortion are seen as murder since life begins at conception (Weiss and Basham 1995).

Buddhism is said generally to disapprove of stem cell research because of its destruction of potential life, and "Buddhist monks are forbidden even to dig the soil, lest living beings be harmed" (Gilbert et al. 2005, 253). On the other hand, humans are thought superior to other animals, and animals may be used in research "if they serve a higher end" and are treated with respect (253). Furthermore, "cloning for reproductive purposes . . . does not require destroying the embryo, and so does not in itself violate Buddhist precepts" (Reichardt et al. 2004, 669).

A most interesting comparison of religious and secular views is presented by Ernle W. D. Young, a recently retired professor of philosophy from Stanford University who started life as a theologian. His definitions of *morality* and *ethics* differ from those given in the opening paragraph of this chapter (Young 2001). He says that morality is a religious tradition and that only adherents to the particular faith agree with the religion's vision of the highest good, whereas ethics is a secular view using public language and reason and appeal to shared societal values. Thus "ethics is more at home than morality with uncertainty and ambiguity. Moral systems tend to see things in terms of right and wrong, black-and-white" (163). For this reason, says Young, he made a conscious decision early in his professional life to teach philosophical ethics rather than theological morality.

ETHICAL ISSUES FOR STEM CELL RESEARCH

A fundamental ethical issue regarding scientific research is whether there is a right (perhaps a First Amendment right) of "free speech" to do research (President's Council on Bioethics 2004a, 61). This has not been tested in the courts and thus is unsettled legally. Research goals as defined by the National Bioethics Advisory Commission are "to produce health benefits for individuals who are suffering from serious and often fatal diseases" (National Bioethics Advisory Commission 1999, 68).

As with health or medical research generally, the criteria for research—especially with children or vulnerable subjects—are less stringent if there are likely therapeutic benefits. Thus it is argued that research on embryos or fetuses would be justified if the research were likely to benefit the embryos or fetuses themselves. This, of course, does not apply to embryonic stem cell research, which sacrifices the blastocyst. Then the question becomes "Is it justified to sacrifice a blastocyst for the benefit of others—that is, for the benefit of fully developed but ill children or adults?" Indeed, the tension in embryonic stem cell research (or research with adult stem cells modified by SCNT to avoid immunologic rejection) is balancing the destruction of the blastocyst against the potential for understanding, ameliorating, even curing disease. This, of course, is a utilitarian approach. Another concern that must be balanced is the "therapeutic misconception" of the research subject or donor: the belief of the subject that he or she will personally benefit. Therapeutic misconception is obvious and straightforward in research on disorders that research subjects have themselves when that research has not been demonstrated to be efficacious. Therapeutic misconception of egg donors (even of those who may be induced to donate by payment of their IVF expenses, or payment for undergoing ovarian hyperstimulation and oocyte recovery if they are healthy "volunteers") is less obvious and less direct: many healthy individuals have one or more relatives or close friends who have a disease that might be benefited by stem cell therapy, and thus the donor may believe that the research is in the best interest of the relative or friend.

And if the reasonably anticipated benefits of the research justify the research, does it deserve federal (or state) support? Does the research require regulation for which federal support would allow high-level oversight (as is customary with research funded by the National Institutes of Health [NIH])? Indeed, how should stem cell research be financed, overseen, and reported? Is oversight inadequate with private rather than public funding? Will private investors be willing to support research that is not highly likely to generate a substantial profit within several years? Will rare disorders be studied at all if research is funded privately rather than supported publicly?

It would be unnecessary to use embryonic stem cells if adult or multipotent stem cells were adequate for the research or for a treatment to be undertaken. Karen Lebacqz of the Pacific School of Religion and the Graduate Theological Union in Berkeley, California, believes that it is permissible to use early embryos in research but that one must minimize harm: she states that if one can do the research without destroying the blastocyst, that should be a goal. Some might say that to perform research on human embryos or pre-embryos is to devalue them. Professor Lebacqz, however, states that to use an embryo in research is not to devalue and disrespect it; researchers respect autonomous persons by providing informed consent, respect sentient beings by limiting pain and fear, and can respect the embryo simply by limiting the way in which it is manipulated and how one speaks about it (Lebacqz 2001).

Embryonic stem cells for research will probably come largely from blastocysts from cryopreserved embryos stored in IVF clinics and otherwise destined to be discarded because the couple no longer wishes to have further children. In 2002 a Society for Assisted Reproductive Technology (SART) and Rand survey of 430 assisted reproductive technology practices estimated that there were nearly four hundred thousand such frozen embryos in the United States (Hoffman et al. 2003), and approximately four embryos are frozen with each cycle of IVF (Klock 2004). Many of these embryos would eventually be discarded rather than used by the parents or given up for adoption by another infertile couple. No one would argue that there need not be fully informed, voluntary consent for donation of embryos or eggs, but should consent for their use in research be obtained only from the woman or should it be obtained from the couple if the donation is of an embryo? Can there be financial incentives for donation? IVF is very expensive, and payment for donation or reduced fees could partially offset the expense. A questionnaire to directors of 341 American IVF clinics revealed that "the disposal of human embryos created in excess in American IVF clinics varies in ways suggesting both moral sensitivity and ethical convergence" (Gurmankin et al. 2004). Most health care professionals in assisted reproductive technology agree with the American Society of Reproductive Medicine that women or couples with frozen embryos should decide whether to store them (or continue to store them) for their own future reproductive purposes before considering whether to donate them (whether to another couple or for research). And if they are to donate for research, they should know the nature and purpose of the research, and consent should be obtained by someone other than the fertility specialist (Ethics Committee, American Society for Reproductive Medicine 2002).

The preceding discussion relates to embryos created in excess of those either used by an infertile couple or donated to another infertile couple. IVF and other assisted reproductive techniques do not solve the problem of all infertile couples. Thus donation of eggs (and sperm) has become a business such that young women with socially desirable features are not infrequently paid many thousands of dollars for undergoing ovarian hyperstimulation and oocyte recovery. There is not only a risk of the hyperstimulation syndrome (which may require hospitalization and can even be fatal), and at least a theoretical possibility that hyperstimulation might cause cancer, but also clearly the danger of exploitation of poor women. Under certain experimental conditions embryonic stem cells can sometimes be induced to form what appear to be oocytes, and hopefully this may lessen dependence upon egg donors (Gilbert et al. 2005).

Perhaps the biggest ethical issue regarding stem cell research from a utilitarian perspective is the potential missed opportunity if restrictions on research preclude (or even just delay) research that might lead to cures (or even just amelioration) of diseases thought to be amenable to the promise of stem cell therapy. And from a public policy perspective, failure to enact enabling legislation or regulation, thereby allowing the status quo to persist, is de facto a policy decision.

Although the news was of lesser potential overall impact than delay of embryonic stem cell research and knowledge not obtained, the entire scientific research community was shocked to learn the reports of the Korean scientist Woo Suk Hwang were fraudulent. He had reported that his laboratory had produced patient-specific human embryonic stem cell lines by SCNT and that this could be accomplished with remarkable efficiency (Hwang, Ryu, et al. 2004; Hwang, Roh, et al. 2005; Snyder and Loring 2006). This is not an ethical issue in the sense of a dilemma: that is, it is not an issue with two arguably justifiable, though opposing, alternatives. Rather, this fabrication is outright scientific misconduct. In addition, multiple authors provided inadequate accountability for the reports. And to add insult to injury, oocytes had been obtained from junior scientists in Hwang's laboratory, raising concerns of actual or potential coercion. A coauthor admitted to paying for egg donation (without notifying Hwang), and it is reported that the serious risks of egg donation were not explained to all those who donated and that sixteen of one hundred donors required treatment in the hospital (Cho et al. 2006).

Although it is doubly sad that a controversial field of high-expectation research should be tainted by such abhorrent behavior, as Snyder and Loring (2006) emphasize, the irregularities were "unveiled by the scientific community itself" (322), and "it is critically important . . . that the response to the Hwang scandal not include the imposition of levels of untutored government regulation, draconian legislation, or criminalization" (333). Furthermore, in the wake of its embarrassment, "South Korea is more determined than ever to become a force in worldwide stem cell research." In addition to increased ethical standards, a task force of scientists and public officials expects the South Korean government "to spend $454 million over the next 10 years" (Normile 2006, 1298). Yet another potential contributor is China. Murray and Spar (2006) state, "Stem-cell research in China is unlikely ever to be prone to the intense moral politicking that characterizes the field in the West." They ask, "Is China—like Korea, perhaps, and Singapore—poised to participate in the next round of global scientific advances?" (1192).

ETHICAL ISSUES FOR STEM CELL THERAPY

Whereas bone marrow transplantation and more recently infusion of adult stem cells (obtained from cord blood or from pheresis of cells from the circulation of HLA-matched donors) have been performed successfully for years, therapy with embryonic stem cells is in its infancy. It must be considered experimental, and at a minimum—unless autologous stem cells are obtained—there is risk of immunologic rejection and thus risk of complications from drugs used for purposeful immunosuppression. There is also risk of graft-versus-host disease, and the opponents of embryonic stem cell research are quick to point out that stem cells injected subcutaneously in animals sometimes cause teratoma formation, a serious theoretical risk that enthusiasts believe unlikely. Further, a serious potential problem for stem cell research and therapy limited to use of the cell lines produced prior to the August 9, 2001, pronouncement by President George W. Bush is that all were grown on a medium containing bovine serum and mouse feeder cells, raising concern of cross-species transfer of infection and perhaps immunologic concerns as well (Dawson et al. 2003; Committee on Guidelines 2005).

Another serious potential problem for all research in which the subjects are patients is that of the therapeutic misconception, the overly optimistic expectation of therapeutic benefit on the part of a subject of research of unproven therapeutic benefit. Indeed, all embryonic stem cell therapy at this time must be considered experimental (research), but the diseases for which stem cell therapy may be useful are so severe that many patients demand to be subjects, believing that they will benefit or that the experimental "treatment" is their only option. The hype of unethical investigators or charlatans is so seductive that there are unrealistic expectations, and there are subjects who are being misled, abused, and pauperized, even today.

Another ethical issue is the use of stem cell research to enhance human traits and characteristics. Although there may be no sharp dividing line between trait and disease, there appears to be public consensus that stem cell research should be applied only to the treatment of disease.

A future but enormously important issue is, Who will have access to the benefits of research and eventually of therapy? And at what expense? Currently, there is a lack of ethnic and racial diversity in the available stem cell lines (just as there is lack of access to IVF because of the substantial cost of treatment for infertility). Stem cell lines should be created for racial equity and for rare disorders.

ETHICAL ISSUES FOR PUBLIC POLICY REGULATION OF STEM CELL RESEARCH AND THERAPY

IVF, whose development for the treatment of infertility raised many of the ethical issues we now face in stem cell research (in part because "spare" cryopreserved embryos are a major potential source of stem cells), was first clinically successful in Great Britain with the birth of Louise Brown in 1978 under the tutelage of Drs. Robert Edwards and Patrick Steptoe. Edwards, who had experimentally fertilized a human egg in vitro in 1969, invited Steptoe (who provided expertise in the laparoscopic recovery of oocytes) to join him in the treatment of infertile couples, and the second couple they treated gave birth to Louise Brown.[3] Despite Edwards's extraordinary attention to ethical issues, the resultant public concern led to the appointment in Great Britain of the Warnock Committee in 1982 to "examine the social, ethical, and legal implications" of assisted reproductive technology. Their influential report (Warnock 1985/1992, 4) led to the Human Fertilization and Embryology Act of 1990, which allowed embryo research to the fourteenth day or to the development of the primitive streak, after which investigators could not "keep or make use of a human IVF embryo" (Human Fertilization and Embryology Authority 2003, 94). Some found this anomalous in the sense that once the embryo developed to the point of a fundamental increase in moral status, it was to be destroyed or discarded.

Assuming that we agree that treatment of infertility is desirable and that research in reproductive technology and research of embryonic as well as adult stem cells should be pursued, the critical questions are "How should they be funded?" and "How should they be regulated?" In 1994 the NIH appointed the Human Embryonic Research Panel, which closely followed the provisions of the British Human Fertilization and Embryology Act in recommending federal funding of research on embryos up to the appearance of the primitive streak or to fourteen days following conception, whichever came first. Interestingly, it also recommended forbidding cloning by nuclear transfer.

The basic question for us in the United States is how in a pluralistic society we should develop necessary public policy regarding ethically contested matters. There must be respect for minority opinion, but the minority should not hold the entire public hostage to its personal or idiosyncratic values (Childress 2004). Recently the position that we should prohibit stem cell research (because destruction of the embryo to obtain stem cells is equivalent to killing an innocent person) even though it might benefit others has been called the "embryoist objection," and those who hold the position "embryoists" (Liao 2005, 9). As concluded by the Committee on Guidelines for Human Embryonic Stem Cell Research of the National Academies (i.e., of the National Research Council and the Institute of Medicine), ethical concern should not prohibit stem cell research but rather should require regulation and oversight (Committee on Guidelines 2005). This is a practical conclusion of our need to strike an acceptable balance between the ethical concerns and the promise of stem cell research and therapy (the two matters of societal agreement that are in conflict). To strike an acceptable balance or compromise and to find common understandings has been complicated by the politicization of the issues by the president (Stolberg 2006) and the sound-bite mentality of the media, which converts the nuanced gray of ethical reflection into black-and-white opinions (Kahn 2006).

Appreciating these concerns, President George W. Bush, in an August 9, 2001, public announcement on "an issue that is one of the most profound of our time" (though it would soon be overshadowed by, if not forgotten because of, the events of September 11, 2001), compromised by allowing federal funding of research using stem cell lines that had been derived, via private funds, for reproductive purposes (if donors had given informed consent without financial inducement) and that had already been in existence as of August 9, 2001 (Bush 2001a; President's Council on Bioethics 2004a, 181). However, he did not allow using any that might be created subsequently (because doing so would allow funding of studies that required destruction of human life, blastocysts, to obtain stem cells) (Committee on Guidelines 2005). The president's decision is hailed by supporters as a reasonable compromise, but many people are disappointed: some from the far right feel that even the compromise encourages the destruction of human life, and others from the left believe that the restriction will delay—if not preclude—research and therapy. Thus President Bush's compromise has not satisfied either side of the debate on either ethical or pragmatic grounds, and it is increasingly seen as unduly restrictive of research, since the more than sixty to seventy lines of approved stem cells thought to be in existence at that time have dwindled to less than two dozen, and these lack genetic and disease diversity and cannot be used for human therapy because they were grown in bovine serum and on mouse feeder cells that risk the transmission of animal viruses. Although recent congressional legislation would have permitted human embryonic stem cell production and research, a July 19, 2006, presidential veto continues to restrict federal funding to lines produced prior to August 9, 2001. The President's Council on Bioethics (2004a, 63–73) summarized arguments critical of the president's 2001 compromise in three categories:

1. Arbitrary: The cutoff date is capricious and not morally relevant. If the research is immoral (because it requires destruction of human life), it should be prohibited, not simply not funded. Furthermore, it should be prohibited in the private, not just the public, sector (Sandel 2004).

2. Unsustainable: If effective therapy is achieved with the results of embryonic stem cell research, the public pressure for expanded research will be overwhelming. If the approved cell lines are inadequate for learning what might be learned without the

restriction, the policy should be changed (before scientists leave the United States to carry out their research abroad in Europe or Asia).

3. Inconsistent: The policy makes inconsistent distinctions: between what is funded and what is permitted, between what is permitted (research with the previously created cell lines) and what is not (the destruction of blastocysts to obtain stem cells in order to create new stem cell lines), and between investigators who are complicit and those who are not.

Limiting public funding and relying on private investment was noted already five years ago (National Bioethics Advisory Committee 1999, iv) to have the potential to "severely limit scientific and clinical progress." And recently in the *Washington Post* on August 23, 2004, Ruth Faden and John Gearhart of Johns Hopkins University wrote that "current policy is substantially retarding progress in stem cell research" (A15).

It is important to appreciate that President Bush's "compromise" and the restriction of NIH funding of embryonic stem cell research to lines created prior to August 9, 2001, did not mark the beginning of ethical and public policy concerns about embryonic research: as stated above, recommendations limiting such research were made in the United Kingdom in 1982 by the Warnock Committee and in 1994 by the NIH Human Embryonic Research Panel. Since 1990 fertility treatment and embryo research in the United Kingdom has been regulated by the Human Fertilization and Embryology Authority. The NIH panel in 1994 also recommended forbidding cloning by nuclear transfer!

Public Law 105–78, 513 (a), the Dickey-Wicker Amendment or rider to all annual appropriations since 1996 (Daley 2004) for the Department of Health and Human Services (of which the NIH is a part), forbids the use of funds to support research "in which a human embryo [is] destroyed, discarded, or knowingly subjected to risk of injury greater than that allowed for fetuses in utero." The human embryo is defined as "any organism . . . that is derived by fertilization, parthenogenesis [development from an unfertilized, usually female, gamete], cloning or other means from one or more human gametes or human diploid cells" (National Bioethics Advisory Commission 1999). The Dickey Amendment is simplistically epitomized as "a don't fund, don't ban law" (President's Council on Bioethics 2004b, 26).

To keep our discussion of public policy in historical perspective, we should note that it was in 1997 that Ian Wilmut et al. (1997) reported the birth of Dolly the sheep, a product of reproductive cloning (transfer of the nucleus of a somatic udder cell into an oocyte, which was then implanted in a sheep uterus). And it was in 1998 that James Thomson and colleagues reported the recovery of embryonic stem cells from a human blastocyst and that, in the same issue of *Science,* John Gearhart reported embryonic germ cells from an aborted human fetus (Thomson et al. 1998; Gearhart 1998; Donovan 1994, 1998).

NIH director Harold Varmus asked the General Counsel for the Department of Health and Human Services whether the NIH might provide federal funds for human embryonic stem cell research that used stem cells from embryos left over from IVF. He was informed that the omnibus appropriations rider did not preclude such funding for such research "because the cells themselves do not meet the statutory, medical, or biological definition of a human embryo" (National Bioethics Advisory Commission 1999, 35). Thus, although the statute "prohibits federal funding for research in which a human embryo is actually destroyed," it apparently does not prohibit "funding of research that depends upon the prior destruction of a human embryo [i.e., using stem cells recovered using private funds, since] the statute defines embryos as 'organisms,' and stem cells are not organisms and therefore are not embryos" (National Bioethics Advisory Commission 2000, D6). However, "General Counsel did not [specifically] address the question of whether the statute prohibits federal funding of research that is dependent on the prior destruction of a human embryo" (D6).

At question also, of course, is the legislative intent. Representative Jay Dickey himself wrote that the amendment "prevents federal funding of destructive experiments on live human embryos" (Dickey 1995, A27). Furthermore, congressional members of the Appropriations Committee raised concern that the Dickey Amendment might prevent progress in research, and in 1999 the committee urged the NIH "to give full consideration to a grant proposal for a stem cell biology center ... which would further research in embryonic stem cell biology" (National Bioethics Advisory Commission 2000, D8). However, "there is no indication that either the proponents or the opponents contemplated the situation ... in which research that destroyed the embryo was separately conducted from research using the cells derived from the embryo." Nevertheless, "DHHS reasonably determined that the prohibition on federal funding of human embryo research does not prohibit federal funding of research using pluripotent stem cells derived from an embryo provided that those cells are derived without the support of federal funds" (D8).

Several commentators have detailed the inadequacies of the stem cell sources to which researchers dependent on federal funding are currently restricted. According to Faden and Gearhart (2004, A15), "No non-embryonic sources of stem cells . . . have been shown to have anything like the potential to lead to viable treatments for such diseases as juvenile diabetes, Parkinson's, and spinal cord injury that stem cells derived from very early embryos do." The authors go on to say that "[t]he embryonic stem cell lines the President approved for federal funding, all of which were derived before August 2001, are clearly inadequate to advance stem cell science. There are too few of them, no more than 21. All . . . risk mouse viruses. . . . There are just too few cell lines to even begin to accommodate the genetic diversity of our population." According to Faden et al. (2003), "[u]nless the problem of biological access is carefully addressed, an American stem cell bank may end up benefiting primarily white Americans, to the relative exclusion of the rest of the population" (3). They comment that "[t]he burdens of ensuring a just system of access to stem cell therapies will fall disproportionately on women relative to men (for whom gamete donation is, by comparison, inconsequential). . . . A related challenge will be securing sufficient gamete donations from minority populations and, in particular, from African Americans" (12). Furthermore, embryos created for IVF will not have sufficient genetic and health/disease diversity, and thus there will be a need for embryos created to obtain stem cells for research and therapy—whether by egg and sperm donation or by SCNT (Gilbert et al. 2005). "Most of the available cell lines are owned by private companies, and the nine cell lines that are publicly available are not suitable for human trials: Many are beginning to show signs of genetic instability, and all were grown in the potentially contaminating presence of mouse 'feeder' cells" (Philpott 2005, 1). Finally, there are no disease stem cell lines for research of diseases. In 2003 only $25 million was allocated for embryonic stem cell research, whereas $190.7 million was spent on research with less promising adult stem cells (Faden and Gearhart 2004).

These concerns have led politicians to continue pressing for reduced federal restrictions on funding embryonic stem cell research. In May 2006, one year after passage of the House bill (HR 810), forty Democrats urged Senate Majority Leader Bill Frist, MD, to allow a Senate vote (Capitol Health Call 2006). On July 18, 2006, the Stem Cell Research Enhancement Act of 2005 passed in the Senate by 63 to 37 (four votes short of the two-thirds majority required to override a presidential veto). As anticipated, the president vetoed the bill the following day

(Schwartz and Rae 2006), and the House vote (235–193) was 51 votes short of the two-thirds required to override (Stolberg 2006). Nevertheless, one anticipates the restrictions will delay, not prevent, scientific progress.

Whereas federal funding of research allows high-level NIH peer review for funding approval of proposed research and requires IRB approval and oversight of ongoing research, privately funded research need only comply with state and federal law. In November 2004, well before the presidential veto of the legislation that would have permitted federal funding of research on embryonic stem cell lines created after the arbitrary August 9, 2001, date, voters of the state of California, by a comfortable margin of 59 percent, approved Proposition 71, the California Stem Cell Research and Cures Act (a statewide ballot initiative that provides $3 billion over ten years preferentially for stem cell research not eligible for federal funding), which established the California Institute of Regenerative Medicine (CIRM). The Scientific and Medical Accountability Standards Working Group (which reports to an Independent Citizens Oversight Committee) has drafted ethical guidelines largely incorporating those of the National Academy of Sciences but with additional emphasis on the donation, consent, and procurement of oocytes; the protection of oocyte donors; and donors' preferences regarding use of their gametes, embryos, or somatic cells (CIRM 2006b). California's initiative was challenged legally, and despite a Superior Court ruling that the proposition is constitutional in its entirety (CIRM 2006a), the plaintiffs may appeal. Anticipating resolution of the legal challenges, consistent with the legislation that allowed bridge financing by bond anticipation notes, private philanthropists have provided $14 million (to be repaid only if litigation is resolved in the state's favor) and may provide another $30 million, and on July 20, the day after President Bush's July 19, 2006, veto, Governor Schwarzenegger ordered a loan of $150 million (nearly four times the NIH budget for human embryonic stem cell research) (Romney 2006). Thus state support of human embryonic stem cell research appears to be required for the immediate future and has been approved in Connecticut, Illinois, Maryland, and New Jersey—though in relatively small amounts compared with California (Romney 2006).

As discussed in a subsequent section in greater detail, in 2005 the National Academy of Sciences recommended voluntary guidelines based upon the belief that human embryonic stem cell research should not be prohibited but requires regulation and oversight. For the latter it recommended institutional or regional human embryonic stem cell research oversight (ESCRO) committees and a national committee to monitor the guidelines and provide a forum for discussion of stem cell research issues.

Of international significance, in March 2005 the General Assembly adopted the United Nations Declaration on Human Cloning, which "prohibits all forms of human cloning [therapeutic as well as reproductive] in as much as they are incompatible with human dignity and the protection of human life" (Devolder and Savulescu (2006, 7). Devolder and Savulescu (2006) believe there is a moral imperative to conduct embryonic stem cell and cloning research. Therapeutic cloning (SCNT) is important because we should do more rather than fewer transplants (e.g., for cardiac disease) and therapeutic cloning might allow for histocompatible transplants. Therapeutic cloning is also important to study diseases in vitro (cellular models of disease), to test drugs in vitro, to study the influence of genes upon drug action and mechanisms thereof, and to study cell growth and differentiation (which may allow us to learn how to transdifferentiate and dedifferentiate cells and to understand malignancy). In fact, the authors believe that therapeutic cloning is so important that "[t]he United Nations must immediately retract its misguided and immoral Declaration on Human Cloning before it consigns many more future people to early and avoidable suffering and death" (19) The authors respond to the many objections to therapeutic cloning: that it destroys potential human life, that availability of adult stem cells makes SCNT unnecessary, that therapeutic cloning is a slippery slope to reproductive cloning, that the technique would be unaffordable for many, that it may be unsafe, and that it may exploit women. To promote community understanding and acceptance of therapeutic cloning and research, they recommend transparency of research, independent oversight and periodic review, public and legislative control, respect for the diversity of values, and reassurance and demonstration of benefit.

A fascinating, but currently only theoretical, public policy question may face us in the future if stem cells allow for life extension (increasing the duration of human life) or age retardation (slowing down the process of senescence). Theoretically, stem cells may have the potential for both (Gilbert et al. 2005). In turn, this could potentially not only change human aspirations (would one still wish to have children?) but also lead to an economic crisis (with wealth concentrated in the "healthy elderly").

Another extremely important public policy and legal issue for all biomedical research is the problematic "patentability of nature." With regard to human embryonic stem cell research, it is important to note that the Wisconsin Alumni Research Foundation owns two patents for "Primate Embryonic Stem Cells," including human embryonic stem cells. These patents could "exclude everyone else in the United States from making, using, selling, offering for sale, or importing any human embryonic stem cells . . . until 2015. The US patent law allows claims to a 'form' not found in nature, so claims for an 'isolated' or 'purified' preparation are acceptable" (Loring and Campbell 2006, 1716). The Wisconsin Foundation could "license others to practice the patented invention in exchange for royalties [, and] currently WARF requires a license agreement for distribution of any human embryonic stem cell lines in the United States" (1717). The current charge is $500 for academic investigators but $125,000 initially and $40,000 annually for a commercial license. The patents are in legal contention ("request for interference"), and "the outcome of this case may have important consequences for embryonic stem cell researchers, funding agencies, and companies" (1717).

CAN SCIENCE RESOLVE THE ETHICAL DILEMMAS AND THE PUBLIC POLICY DEBATE?

In this section I describe seven scientific approaches that have been proposed to resolve the ethical dilemma and public policy debate by avoiding the sacrifice of the blastocyst to obtain stem cells. The President's Council on Bioethics in May 2005 published a white paper entitled "Alternative Sources of Human Pluripotent Stem Cells." It describes and analyzes (from an ethical, scientific, and pragmatic or practical perspective) four of five approaches discussed by the council on December 3, 2004. Another of the approaches described here (and also mentioned by Chairman Kass at the council meeting on December 3, 2004; see President's Council on Bioethics 2004a, session 6), the parthenogenetic approach, was only briefly described in the white paper, perhaps because on further reflection it was considered to create but then to destroy or harm human life, which the other four approaches were thought to avoid doing. Another possible reason is that some say the parthenote is not human because it has two maternal sets of chromosomes but no paternal chromosomes, and Kass stated, "There's an almost certainty that this will not go on—could not go on—to develop into a child" (President's Council on Bioethics 2004a, session 6).

In December 2004 the Reproductive Genetics Institute reported in Reproductive Biomedicine Online that one cell (a blastomere) can be removed from the early morula (just as it is in preimplantation genetic diagnosis [PGD]—which suggests this approach is not really new after all) without destruction of the pre-embryo and that the single cell can be cultured into a line of stem cells for therapeutic research (Strelchenko et al. 2004; Pearson 2006). The remaining cells of the morula could develop into an embryo and fetus apparently without defect, thus seemingly—at least at first glance—avoiding the issue of destruction of the blastocyst and the religious and ethical concern that this engenders. However, since the cell that is removed from the morula is totipotent or at least pluripotent and thus could develop into an embryo and fetus, one still has the problem of thwarting potential human life—that is, sacrificing what could have become a person. Furthermore, if in the future we could dedifferentiate adult stem cells or conceivably somatic (body) cells so that they could become totipotent (or even just pluripotent), then sacrificing an adult stem cell or a body cell would be tantamount to killing a potential person and what some would call "murder"!

This approach (of removing one blastomere from the early morula to produce a line of stem cells without destroying the blastocyst) is just one of seven approaches recently proposed and discussed to obtain stem cells for research or therapy by what some consider to be an "ethically acceptable" technique (and others consider to be self-deception). A second approach was reported in the *Boston Globe* on November 21, 2004: William B. Hurlbut, MD, PhD, a Stanford professor of neurology and neurological science who has also studied theology and medical ethics (Cook 2004) and who is a member of the President's Council on Bioethics, has proposed altering ("jinxing") DNA of the nucleus of an adult cell before it is implanted into an enucleated egg (SCNT, which Hurlbut pejoratively calls therapeutic cloning) in such a way that the blastocyst could not become a fetus or child. Techniques to accomplish this were proposed in 2002 by independent scientists in the United States and Germany, and Hurlbut's contribution is to use this scientific information to "reframe the moral argument" (Holden and Vogel 2004, 2174). And recently inactivation of a gene (Cdx2) necessary for development of the trophoblast and for axial development and organization of the embryo in mice has been reported (Chawengsaksophak et al. 2004). Thus a blastocyst would form (whose viable inner cells could be harvested to grow a stem line) whose outer cells could not form a trophoblast and placenta, so that the inner cells, even if not harvested, could not become a fetus or child.

Hurlbut analogizes this scientific approach to the rare condition in nature in which an oocyte (egg) in a woman forms a tumor, a hydatidiform mole or teratoma, that may form limb and organ primordia, even hair and teeth, but not a fetus. The lack of a coherent structure or integrated organization of the teratoma in nature or of the blastocyst from altered nuclear transfer precludes the development of an embryo or organism, and thus the use of cells from the mass is said not to be the destruction of human life.

Indeed, there was great interest in the approach when discussed on December 3, 2004, by the President's Council on Bioethics (President's Council on Bioethics 2004a; Brown 2004; Saletan 2004). But Melton, Daley, and Jennings, in their critique of the proposal in the December 30, 2004, *New England Journal of Medicine,* state that it is not known whether human embryos deficient in the gene would "die at the same stage as mice" deficient in the gene and that the stem cells might well be abnormal and thus of limited "usefulness in research and clinical applications" (2791). Responding to this latter objection, Hurlbut suggests that one could restore the inactivated gene in order to normalize the stem cells (2791). But Melton et al. argue that the "ethical superiority of altered nuclear transfer rests on a flawed scientific assumption" (2791). The flaw is that, in their opinion, it is no more morally acceptable to destroy a gene-mutant embryo than to destroy a normal embryo—that the moral status of an embryo is not dependent upon the gene that it lacks or whose mutant it possesses. Furthermore, they believe, as do many others in contrast to Hurlbut, that it is justified "to use preimplantation-stage human embryos in a search to understand human biology and cure serious diseases" (2792).

A third major technique to mitigate ethical concern in the recovery of embryonic stem cells was presented to the President's Council on Bioethics on December 3, 2004: that of Donald Landry and Howard Zucker (2004) of Columbia University. They state that "up to 60% of the embryos created for invitro fertilization (IVF) treatment are considered 'nonviable'—meaning development has been arrested but individual cells are still functioning" (quoted in Holden and Vogel 2004, 2176). They analogize that since it is permissible to obtain organs for transplantation from "brain-dead" humans, it should be acceptable to obtain stem cells from developmentally "arrested" or organismically "dead" embryos. They believe chemical or genetic markers can be found to reliably diagnose "the irreversible arrest of cell division," which they consider "death" of the embryo. Further, they note several studies that suggest "some prospect for producing normal cells from dead embryos" (President's Council on Bioethics 2004a), but whether healthy stem cell lines can be achieved remains to be demonstrated. Once again, ethically, if the cells obtained could become healthy differentiated tissues, why might they not be differentiated to form an entire organism, a fetus? An approach analogous to that of Landry and Zucker has recently been published: Schwartz and Rae (2006) argue that low-grade embryos (low-grade on morphologic or biologic criteria) "might qualify for stem cell harvest [if] suitable high-grade embryos" exist for implantation (773). "Although technical advances have made it possible to implant low-grade embryos, their implantation rate is low, their miscarriage rate is high [and] they are usually allowed to die" (772).

At the President's Council on Bioethics in December 2004, Chairman Leon Kass noted a fourth technique, "another morally non-problematic route . . . to getting new embryonic stem cell lines" (President's Council on Bioethics 2004b, session 6), as also reported in the *New Scientist* (Coughlan 2004). By injecting phospholipase c-zeta, an enzyme from sperm, Karl Swann, of the University of Wales, stimulated human eggs to divide (as if they had been fertilized) and to become blastocysts. Swann believes the parthenogenetic blastocysts with two sets of maternal, and no paternal, chromosomes should not be considered "potential human life" (Coughlan 2004).

Peter J. Bryant (pers. comm., Dec. 3, 2004), a developmental cell biologist and a professor at the University of California, Irvine, states if one achieved parthenogenesis "by suppressing the first meiotic division . . . the progeny would be a reproductive clone of the mother" but that if one suppressed the second division, "that generates homozygosity which would be dangerous" because it "would expose recessive deleterious alleles that usually exist in natural populations." Thus he believes "it would be a mistake to try to 'sidestep' the ethical issues by generating and using stem cells that are genetically abnormal."

From an ethical perspective, even though to date "the only mammalian parthenote—a mouse—that has made it to term was the product of heavy genetic intervention" (Holden and Vogel 2004, 2175), how can one be sure that a human parthenote could not become a fetus? If it could, the ethical concern would be that harvesting stem cells from a human parthenote blastocyst would be "killing." Recently in Italy, where creation or destruction of human embryos for research is banned, two investigators (Tiziana Brevini and Fulvio Gandolfi of the University of Milan) reported that they were able to derive two stem cell–like lines from parthenotes created from 104 human eggs ("Human eggs supply 'ethical' stem cells" 2006).

A fifth technique is the so-called Holy Grail of stem cell therapy: reprogramming differentiated cells into dedifferentiated pluripotent stem cells so that they can grow as a stem cell line and be used to repair or replace damaged tissues or organs. This may still be only a scientist's dream, but according to an article in *Science,* "Shinya Yamanaka of Kyoto University . . . reported [at the fourth annual meeting of the International Society for Stem Cell Research, June 29–July 1, 2006] that upregulating just four genes can apparently turn mouse stem cells into cells that closely resemble embryonic stem cells" (Vogel 2006a). This has not yet been done using human skin cells. Nevertheless, it appears to be an important step toward the "Holy Grail." This approach, if confirmed, would avoid not only the need to destroy blastocysts from IVF rejects or leftovers (whether alive or dead) or from SCNT but also the need to obtain donated eggs or embryos; further, it would avoid immunologic incompatibility (Holden and Vogel 2004). However, if the cells were dedifferentiated to totipotency (not just to pluripotency), even this approach would be objectionable to prolife fundamentalists who believe that the dedifferentiated cell could potentially become a human and thus must not be sacrificed. On the other hand, if dedifferentiation were achievable, the logical next step in such thinking would be to believe that no adult cell (such as a skin cell or a gastrointestinal cell, many of which are shed each day) could be discarded because any such cell—ideally handled—could become a baby! This, of course, is a reductio ad absurdum.

I should note a sixth technique, even though it was quite hypothetical or theoretical until recently. It is the subject of one of two target articles on human stem cells in the November–December 2005 issue of the *American Journal of Bioethics* devoted nearly entirely to stem cells. This technique, discovered by S. Matthew Liao of Johns Hopkins, is called the blastocyst transfer method (BTM). Liao (2005) proposed extracting "just enough pluripotent human embryonic stem cells from the inner cell mass to create a cell line, but without harming the embryo's chance of developing into a healthy functioning individual" (11). He admits the "method faces some technical challenges: First, the cells of the inner cell mass . . . at the five-day stage become quite tight and our present technique is not sophisticated enough to extract the cells without destroying the embryo. Second, to create a stable cell line [requires] around 200 human embryonic stem cells" (11–12). In the June 29, 2006, issue of *Nature* it is reported that Takumi Takeuchi and colleagues of Cornell University have derived stem cell lines from one-hundred-cell mouse embryos. This technique might be ethically acceptable to obtain human stem cells (presumably multipotent rather than pluripotent, as in the first of these "ethically acceptable" techniques, which utilized a single blastomere from the four- to eight-cell morula) if the embryo were to survive and to be healthy. Indeed, since the cells would be multipotent rather than pluripotent, this technique would avoid the double-talk that because the three to seven cells not removed from the four- to eight-cell morula in the first technique could go on to develop a healthy embryo and fetus, the PGD-like technique would not involve "killing" a potential life. However, in Takeuchi's experience thus far, the removal of cells from the hundred-cell mouse embryo resulted in a 50 percent mortality.

Finally, I must add a seventh technique for the production of cells that have at least some of the qualities of embryonic stem cells without sacrifice of a blastocyst (indeed, without even involving an embryo). Cells that the German scientists Gerd Hasenfuss and Wolfgang Engel call multipotent adult germline stem cells (maGSCs) were cultured from sperm precursor cells (spermatogonia), as just recently reported on March 24, 2006, in *Nature* (Holden 2006; Guan et al. 2006). The cells differentiated into multiple types of cells of all three germ layers, demonstrating multipotency if not pluripotency. Most recently five additional sources or types of stem cells have been reported but will require peer-reviewed publication and reproducibility in other laboratories (Holden 2007a, 2007b, 2007c).

THE POSSIBLE ACHIEVEMENT OF SOCIETAL CONSENSUS AND THE ADOPTION OF GUIDELINES TO REGULATE AND PROVIDE OVERSIGHT FOR STEM CELL RESEARCH AND THERAPY

A few weeks before his August 9, 2001, compromise policy statement, President George W. Bush said that his policy "would need to balance value and respect for life with the promise of science and hope of saving life" (Bush 2001b). The compromise statement (allowing federally funded research on the approximately sixty to seventy stem cell lines thought to be in existence as of August 9, 2001, but not on any lines that might be developed thereafter) allows us, the president said, "to explore the promise and potential of stem cell research without crossing a fundamental moral line by providing taxpayer funding that would sanction or encourage further destruction of human embryos that have at least the potential for life" (Bush 2001a). According to Chairman Leon Kass, in his opening remarks at the first meeting of the President's Council on Bioethics on January 17, 2002, "[L]eading scientists have indicated that, at least for the research phase (that is, the preclinical phase) of these investigations, the number of embryonic stem cell lines are more than adequate to explore their therapeutic potential" (Kass 2002). He pointed out the irony that both sides of the ethical debate invoked "the principle that calls for protecting, preserving, and saving human life. . . . [The] two sorts of 'vitalists' differed only with respect to whose life mattered most: living, sick children and adults facing risks of decay and premature death, or living human embryos who must be directly destroyed in the process of harvesting their stem cells for research."

Christopher Reeve, frustrated not only by his own quadriplegia but equally by what he perceived as obstruction of scientific research, said, "To opponents of stem cell research, I say spend one hour in a wheelchair. . . . Who are we if we do not use our best knowledge and technology to help someone? It is time to harness the power of government and move forward" (Reeve 2004). In a similar vein, Dustin Hoffman asked, "Do we have to be afflicted to be enlightened?" (Bruck 2002, 82).

A staff working paper for the October 2003 meeting of the President's Council on Bioethics concluded, "The rich and growing ethical debates do suggest the possibility of progress towards greater understanding, and more informed public decision-making" (President's Council on Bioethics 2003). But R. Alta Charo, a professor of law and bioethics at the University of Wisconsin Schools of Law and Medicine, has said that we must recognize that "the substantive conflict . . . cannot be resolved in a manner that is satisfactory to all" (Charo 1995, quoted in Siegel 2000, J9). And Ernle W. D. Young has said, "I am not at all confident that there will be any evidence of mutual tolerance for opposing points of view on this sensitive issue simply because of the difference between [secular] ethics and [religious] morality" (Young 2001, 174).

These views are a mixture of optimism and pessimism, and I must admit that I am both optimistic and pessimistic. We must have public discussion, not debate. We must be tolerant of the views of others and treat others with respect even if we disagree with their views. As Rodney King asked during the Watts riots in Los Angeles in 1992, "Can't we all just get along?" (King 1992).

For those with an absolutist deontologic belief that human individuality or personhood with full moral status begins at conception, there may be no satisfactory solution (unless they are willing to accept one or more of the seven scientific techniques, described above, that have been devised to obtain stem cells in an "ethically acceptable" way). Nevertheless, they might be willing to consider that the majority in society (who have qualitatively or quantitatively different views) have the right to permit human embryonic stem cell research and therapy, though not require it of those who are opposed. This seems particularly reasonable since the vast majority of excess IVF embryos are destined for destruction if they are not donated for adoption.

And for those with a utilitarian perspective who are currently not convinced that the ethical concerns are adequately counterbalanced by the promise of stem cell therapy, perhaps they would agree to continued research with embryonic stem cells (even with human embryonic stem cells), deferring a decision to allow therapy (other than clinical trials) until such time as the evidence convincingly demonstrates benefit for human disease. If they are not willing to agree to continued research with human embryonic stem cells (including experimental clinical trials), hopefully data either with animal embryonic stem cells (for analogous conditions in subhuman animals) or with human adult stem cells will be sufficiently effective to justify research with human embryonic stem cells.

Indeed, in 2001 a National Academies report entitled "Stem Cells and the Future of Regenerative Medicine" (National Research Council/Institute of Medicine 2002) recommended continued research with human embryonic as well as adult stem cells in addition to their derivation by SCNT. Four years later, a National Academies Committee (of the National Research Council's Board on Life Sciences and the Institute of Medicine's Health Science Policy Board) on Guidelines for Human Embryonic Stem Cell Research (cochaired by Jonathan D. Moreno of the University of Virginia and Richard O. Hynes of the Massachusetts Institute of Technology) "did not revisit the debate about whether hES [human embryonic stem] cell research should be pursued" (Committee on Guidelines 2005, 3, 22) and prefaced its report by stating, "[C]oncerns about potential ethical complexities should be cause for judicious oversight and regulation, not necessarily for prohibition" (vii). "It assumed that both hES cell and adult stem cell research would continue in parallel with federal and non-federal funding" (22) and developed "guidelines to encourage responsible practices in hES cell research—regardless of source of funding—including the use and derivation of new stem cell lines derived from surplus blastocysts, from blastocysts produced with donated gametes, or from blastocysts produced using NT [nuclear transfer]" (3). The guidelines "do not cover research with nonhuman stem cells [and] do not apply to reproductive uses of [nuclear transfer]" (4). Further, the committee stated that although "successful resolution of intellectual property issues" would be "critically important in this evolving area of research," it was beyond the committee's charge and capabilities to address adequately all of the legal issues that would arise (22).

These guidelines are so thoughtful and so articulate (showing great sensitivity to opposing religious and philosophical ethical perspectives) that, rather than attempting to review them in detail, I refer the interested reader to them and will simply mention some of the topics covered. The report reviews the history of scientific stem cell discoveries and the history of public policy in embryo and stem cell research, and it lists human embryonic stem cell research priorities and ethical concerns. Some concerns that are not covered in this chapter, but are covered in the report, are the potential consequences of introducing human genes and cells into nonhuman animals (with particular concern for neural and germline tissues in chimeras) and the potential exploitation of women in the recruitment of oocyte donors.

I will not further review the report and its twenty-three specific recommendations except to mention what I consider its two most creative recommendations: First, "[E]ach institution should establish a Human Embryonic Stem Cell Research Oversight (ESCRO) committee. . . . The ESCRO committee would not substitute for an Institutional Review Board but rather would provide an additional level of review and scrutiny warranted by the complex issues raised by hES cell research" (Committee on Guidelines 2005, 107). Second, "A national body should be established to assess periodically the adequacy of the guidelines . . . and to provide a forum for a continuing discussion of the issues involved in hES research" (108). A *New York Times* article of February 16, 2006, reports that the National Academy of Sciences, using private funds, is establishing a national committee "intended to be a standing body that will update the guidelines in the light of new scientific findings and resolve issues too difficult for the local groups" (Wade 2006, A21). In May 2006 the National Academies announced the membership of the committee (cochairs R. Alta Charo of the University of Wisconsin and Richard O. Hynes of MIT) and noted that it is to monitor and revise the guidelines (National Academies 2007a). Indeed, there are now "2007 Amendments to the National Academies' Guidelines for Human Embryonic Stem Cell Research" (Human Embryonic Stem Cell Research Advisory Committee 2007). The Scientific and Medical Accountability Standards Working Group of the California Institute of Regenerative Medicine (CIRM) has already written guidelines in keeping with the National Academies' recommendations. Guidelines have been developed by the American Society of Reproductive Medicine as well as by the National Academies, and

"These guidelines overlap with one another in certain respects and yet conflict in others. . . . This leaves scientific and medical professionals and the nation as a whole with a collection of varying rules for the ethical conduct of stem cell research. Yet for many, the ethical questions raised by stem cell research overshadow the scientific, business, and other issues that surround it and require special attention on the national level" (Cohen, forthcoming).

I believe that the recommendations of the National Academies and the CIRM amply safeguard the public from potential research abuse or misconduct. A tribute to the soundness of the guidelines is their apparently unquestioned acceptance and implementation throughout the United States (with most stem cell research institutes forming, or about to form, human embryonic stem cell research oversight committees). However, many, if not most, of the recommended ESCRO committee functions are prospective, just as are the majority of IRB functions. Indeed, it remains to be seen how the two committees can function in a complementary way (sharing or dividing responsibilities) without unnecessary duplication or delays. I believe there is also need for ongoing (not just prospective) oversight of research, as might be implied by the very name given to the ESCRO committees and by three suggested functions (Committee on Guidelines 2005): first, ESCRO committees "will ensure that US investigators follow standards and procedures" (65); second, "ESCROs and IRBs should require evidence of compliance when protocols are reviewed for renewal" (12); and third, through its ESCRO committee each institution "should establish and maintain a registry of investigators . . . and record descriptive information about the types of research being performed" (48).

The guidelines of the National Academy of Sciences (compliance with which thus far is voluntary rather than mandatory) are not easily adopted globally, but transnational collaboration in research is increasingly feasible and desirable. Thus in February 2006 "over 50 scientists, clinicians, ethicists, journal editors, lawyers, and policymakers from 14 countries convened in Hinxton, Cambridge. . . . [They] articulated a series of normative principles to govern international collaboration in stem cell research . . . [and] made specific recommendations for scientists and journal editors" (Savulescu and Saunders 2006). This consensus statement is to be available at www.hopkinsmedicine.org/bioethics. "The guidelines are consistent with those set out by the US National Academies last year. . . . [They] recommend that certain types of research, such as derivation of new embryonic stem cell lines or generation of chimeric animals, be subject to special review by an independent panel . . . [and] set standards for sharing research materials" (Vogel 2006b). On June 30, 2006, the International Society for Stem Cell Research (ISSCR) presented a draft of "Guidelines for the Conduct of Human Embryonic Stem Cell Research" to its members for comment. The task force acknowledges the guidelines of the National Academy of Science, those of the CIRM, and the consensus statement of the Hinxton Group, as well as the "internationally recognized research ethics guidelines including . . . the Nuremberg Code of 1947, the Declaration of Helsinki of 1964 and 1975, the Belmont Report of 1979, the Council for International Organizations of Medical Science (CIOMS), the International Ethical Guidelines for Biomedical Research Involving Human Subjects of 2002, and the UNESCO Universal Declaration of Bioethics and Human Rights of 2005" (ISSCR 2006, 4). In February 2007 *Science* reported the publication of the ISSCR guidelines and compared them with those of the National Academy of Sciences (Daley et al. 2007). The guidelines are available at www.isscr.org/guidelines/index.htm.

QUESTIONS THE READER MAY ASK

The reader may wish to ask him or herself one or more of the following questions to formulate a personal position on human embryonic stem cell research and therapy:

> Is there a morally significant developmental milestone before which research (on the zygote, the morula, the blastula, the gastrula, the embryo, the pre-viability fetus, the post-viability fetus, the neonate) is justified, and after which it is not? Or, to ask this question in another way: Is conception, the achievement of individual identity, the development of a nervous system, the development of other organs, the appearance of a human form, ensoulment, the achievement of viability, the development of a relationship with its mother, birth, or some further development the morally significant milestone before which research is justified and after which it is not?

> Does the potential of embryonic stem cell therapy to cure disease or replace damaged organs justify destruction of the blastocyst to obtain stem cells for research and/or for therapy?

> Does the immunologic tolerance of stem cells produced by therapeutic cloning (nuclear transfer) justify this technique to obtain genetically near-identical stem cells for therapy?

If the reasonably anticipated promise of embryonic stem cell therapy justifies research on embryonic stem cells, should it be funded only with private funds, with state funds, or with federal funds?

Would ethical oversight of research be different if research funding were private, state, or federal?

Does it matter whether stem cells for research are obtained only from frozen pre-embryos intended to conceive children despite infertility but "left over" because the parents have conceived the number of children they wished from other IVF embryos? Or may investigators use pre-embryos created specifically for research, as now permitted in the United Kingdom by the Human Fertilization and Embryology Authority (Infertility Network 2007)?

What protections are required for potential oocyte donors?

How can one ensure fully informed and voluntary consent for donors and for research subjects, including those with disorders thought to be amenable to stem cell therapy (and thus valid consent subjects who risk the "therapeutic misconception")?

Can there be compensation for donors or reduced fees for IVF therapy for those willing to donate excess embryos for research or for the therapy of other individuals?

How should we protect the rights of those whose views are in the minority? And if a person opposes embryonic stem cell research, will he or she capitulate if research performed elsewhere proves the therapeutic potential? And if not, does one really feel justified in maintaining an absolutist deontologic perspective that precludes embryonic stem cell research and therapy?

OPINIONS OF THE AUTHOR

Even though I will not attempt to answer all the above questions, in fairness I should inform the reader of some of my personal opinions regarding embryonic stem cell research. I believe that the missed opportunity, if we do not allow unfettered human embryonic stem cell research, is so great that we must proceed with embryonic stem cell research (while continuing research with nonembryonic stem cells as well) with the approval of IRBs (and the limited oversight of which they are capable) and the approval (and I hope thorough oversight) of ESCRO committees.

I further believe that the ingenious approaches (removal of one blastomere from a morula; altered nuclear transfer; the use of what has been called a pseudoembryo because of its inability to form a placenta [Liao 2005, 10]; the use of nonviable preembryos; parthenogenesis; and the use of dedifferentiated differentiated cells) do not truly avoid the ethical issues of the conservative, fundamentalist perspective. That is, if one believes that the potential of a cell or cells to develop into a person prohibits their use, the prohibition should be extended to any cells that have this potential, even if other cells (left intact when the cell or cells were taken) may go on to produce a fetus or child. I also believe that the therapeutic use of nonviable pre-embryos is likely to be dangerous or ineffective, though such pre-embryos might be useful for research. On the other hand, the removal of several multipotent stem cells from the inner cell mass of a hundred-cell blastocyst (the "blastocyst transfer method") and—if we ever can achieve it—the dedifferentiation of somatic cells before their differentiation to replace damaged or diseased cells, tissues, or even organs would bypass the ethical objections to destruction of the embryo. In the interim, however, it seems to me unwise to preclude the use of stem cells from healthy blastocysts in stem cell research, if from no other perspective than the utilitarian calculus of the potential therapeutic value of such research. Indeed, I favor the "Third Way" of Lawrence Nelson and Michael Meyer (2005, 33, 36), "a compromise position that recognizes that embryos have some moral worth but still allows for their destruction during the course of respectful experimentation" (Philpott 2005, 2). I believe the National Academies' recommendations are quite sufficient to ensure responsible and ethical human embryonic stem cell research supported by federal funding that would have the added benefit of ensuring high-level oversight of such research.

With regard to the stalemate in public debate and policy, I agree with Christopher Thomas Scott (2006, 186) that "[t]he embryo 'proxy' war—as some politicians and commentators call the conflict encompassing the issues of abortion, in vitro fertilization, and research using embryos and embryonic stem cells—has exacted a toll on American science and medicine." As reported in the *Journal of the American Medical Association,* a review of articles on human embryonic stem cell research published in scientific journals over six years concludes that "contributions from the United States lagged behind those from other countries" (Hampton 2006, 2233; Owen-Smith and McCormick 2006). Scott (2006, 181) comments that "[w]e face great moral hazards here. The first one is choosing ignorance over knowledge, a dangerous precedent for any society. The second one is allowing politics—and politicians—to intrude on the will of a majority of Americans. Third, and most important, is [not] honoring our obligations to those among us who suffer. Our decisions today will determine whether history regards America at the beginning of the 21st century as embarking on a new path of enlightenment or retreating to a dark and pessimistic time."

NOTES

Portions of this chapter appeared in a shorter article of the same title and by the same author (Whittier Law Review 26 (3): 845–68, Spring 2005; copyright 2005 by the Whittier Law Review). This revised manuscript is offered for inclusion in the present volume to complement (and compliment) the exceptionally thoughtful ethical analysis of philosopher Philip J. Nickel from the perspective of a physician and clinical ethicist. It also provides a summary and overview of many of the issues discussed in greater detail in other chapters.

The author is indebted to Irene V. Morris and Anna S. Arietta of the Grunigen Medical Library of the University of California, Irvine for obtaining innumerable articles for the author's review. He is also appreciative of comments on earlier drafts by David L. McArthur, Kristen Renwick Monroe, Philip H. Schwartz, and Jerome S. Tobis.

1. The word *stem*, from the German *stam* and Old English *stemn*, means the main growth of a plant or the trunk of a tree or the end-post of a ship (as in the phrase "from stem to stern"). The meaning of the word *stem* as in *stem cell*, however, dates back only to 1932, when the German phrase *stamen aus* meant "stem from" or "develop from" (Barnhart 1995, 759). *Stemness* is the ability to divide asymmetrically: that is, both to self-renew and to differentiate.

2. For a review more detailed than the brief summary I provide here, please refer to chapter 4 of this book, by Mahtab Jafari, Fanny Elahi, Saba Ozgurt, and Ted Wrigley, "Religious Perspectives on Embryonic Stem Cell Research."

3. Edwards (2005) chronicles not only the science of his research with rabbit blastocysts and stem cells, preimplantation genetic diagnosis, and IVF but his extraordinary attention to the ethical issues.

REFERENCES

Barnhart, Robert K., ed.
   1995. Barnhart Concise Dictionary of Etymology: The Origins of American English Words. New York: HarperCollins.

Bortolotti, L., and J. Harris.
   2006. Embryos and eagles: Symbolic value in research and reproduction. Cambridge Quarterly of Healthcare Ethics 15:22–34.

Brown, D.
   2004. Two stem cell options presented: Human embryos wouldn't be killed. Washington Post, Dec. 4, A1. http://pqasb.pqarchiver.com/washingtonpost/access/752337621.html?dids=752337621:. Accessed Jan. 9, 2007.

Bruck, C.
  2002. Hollywood science: Should a ballot initiative determine the fate of stem
      cell research? New Yorker, Oct. 18, 62–82.
Bush, G. W.
  2001a. President discusses stem cell research. www.whitehouse.gov/news/
      releases/2001/08/print/20010809-2.html. Accessed March 17, 2007.
  2001b. Press conference by President Bush and Italian Prime Minister Berlus-
      coni. www.whitehouse.gov/news/releases/2001/07/print/20010723-3.html.
      Accessed March 22, 2007.
California Institute of Regenerative Medicine.
  2006a. Court upholds constitutionality of stem cell program. Press release,
      April 21. www.cirm.ca.gov/pressreleases/2006/04/04-21-06.asp. Ac-
      cessed Jan. 9, 2007.
  2006b. Third Revised Medical and Ethical Standards Regulations: Notice of
      proposed changes. www.cirm.ca.gov/laws/nopc_stds.asp. July 6. Accessed
      Jan. 10, 2007.
Capitol Health Call.
  2006. Stem cell bill on hold. Journal of the American Medical Association
      295 (22): 2593.
Cascalnho, M., and J. L. Platt.
  2005. New technologies for organ replacement and augmentation. Mayo
      Clinic Proceedings 80 (3): 370–78.
Charo, R. A.
  1995. The hunting of the snark: The moral status of embryos, right-to-lifers,
      and third world women. Stanford Law and Policy Review 6:11–17.
Chawengsaksophak, K., W. deGraph, J. Rossant, J. Deschamps, and F. Beck.
  2004. Cdx2 is essential for axial elongation in mouse development. Proceed-
      ings of the National Academy of Sciences 101 (May 18): 7641–45.
      www.pnas.org/cgi/doi/10.1073/pnas.0401654101. Accessed Jan. 10, 2007.
Childress, J. F.
  2004. Sources of stem cells: Ethical controversies and policy developments in
      the United States. Fetal Diagnosis and Therapy 19:119–23.
Cho, M. K., G. McGee, and D. Magnus.
  2006. Lessons of the stem cell scandal. Science 311 (Feb. 3): 614–15.
Cohen, C. B. Forthcoming. In pursuit of national review of stem cell research. In:
      C. B. Cohen, ed. Reviewing the Stuff of Life: Stem Cells, Ethics, and Public
      Policy, ch. 8. New York: Oxford University Press.
Committee on Guidelines for Human Embryonic Stem Cell Research, Board on
      Life Sciences, National Research Council; Health Sciences Policy Board,
      Institute of Medicine.
  2005. Guidelines for Human Embryonic Stem Cell Research. Washington,
      DC: National Academies Press.
Cook, G.
  2004. New technique eyed in stem cell debate. Boston Globe, Nov. 21.

www.Boston.com/news/nation/articles/2004/11/21/new_technique_eyed_in_stem_cell_debate. Accessed Jan. 10, 2007.

Coughlan, A.
2004. Zapped human eggs divide without sperm. New Scientist, Dec. 1. www.newscientist.com/article.ns?id=dn6733.

Craig, K. D., M. F. Whitfield, R. V. E. Grienau, et al.
1993. Pain in the preterm neonate: Behavioral and physiologic indices. Pain 52:287–99.

Daley, G. Q.
2004. Missed opportunities in embryonic stem-cell research. New England Journal of Medicine 351 (7): 627–28.

Daley, G. Q., et al.
2007. Ethics: The ISSCR guidelines for human embryonic stem cell research. Science 315 (Feb. 2): 603–4.

Dawson, L., A. S. Bateman-House, D. M. Agnew, et al.
2003. Safety issues in cell-based intervention trials. Fertility and Sterility 80 (5): 1077–85.

DeCoppi, P., G. Bartsch, M. M. Siddiqui, et al.
2007. Isolation of amniotic stem cell lines with potential for therapy. Nature Biotechnology 25 (Feb. 1): 100–106.

Dennis, C.
2006. Mining the secrets of the egg. Nature 439 (Feb. 9): 652–55.

Devolder, K., and J. Savulescu.
2006. The moral imperative to conduct embryonic stem cell and cloning research. Cambridge Quarterly of Healthcare Ethics 15:7–21.

Dickey, J.
1995. Lethal experiments. Op-ed. Washington Post, Sept. 29, A27.

Donovan, P. J.
1994. Growth factor regulation of mouse primordial germ cell development. Current Topics in Developmental Biology 29:189–225.
1998. The germ cell: The mother of all stem cells. International Journal of Developmental Biology 42:1043–50.

Edwards, R. G.
2005. Ethics and moral philosophy in the initiation of IVF, preimplantation diagnosis, and stem cells. Reproductive BioMedicine Online 10 (March, suppl. 1): 1–8.

Ethics Advisory Board.
1979. Report and Conclusions: HEW Support of Research Involving Human in Vitro Fertilization and Embryo Transfer. Washington, DC: U.S. Department of Health, Education, and Welfare.

Ethics Committee, American Society for Reproductive Medicine.
2002. Donating spare embryos for embryonic stem-cell research. Fertility and Sterility 78 (5): 957–60.

Evans, M. J., and M. H. Kaufman.
    1981. Establishment in culture of pluripotential cells from mouse embryos.
        Nature 292:154–56.
Faden, R. R., L. Dawson, A. S. Bateman-House, et al.
    2003. Public stem cell banks: Considerations of justice in stem cell research
        and therapy. Hastings Center Report 33 (6): 2–15.
Faden, R. R., and J. D. Gearhart.
    2004. Facts on stem cells. Washington Post, Aug. 23, A15.
Fletcher, J. C.
    2000. Deliberating incrementally on human pluripotential stem cell research.
        In: National Bioethics Advisory Commission, ed. Ethical Issues in Human
        Stem Cell Research, vol. 2, Commissioned Papers. Rockville, MD: Na-
        tional Bioethics Advisory Commission.
Fukuchi, Y., H. Nakajima, D. Sugiyama, I. Hirose, T. Kitamura, and K. Tsuji.
    2004. Human placenta-derived cells have mesenchymal stem/progenitor cell
        potential. Stem Cells 22:649–58.
Gazzaniga, M. S.
    2005. The Ethical Brain. New York: Dana Press.
Gearhart, J. D.
    1998. New potential for human embryonic stem cells. Science 282:1061–62.
Geron Ethics Advisory Board.
    1999. Research with human embryonic stem cells: Ethical considerations.
        Hastings Center Report 29 (2): 31–36.
Gilbert, S. F., A. L. Tyler, and E. J. Zackin.
    2005. Bioethics and the New Embryology: Springboards for Debate. New
        York: W. H. Freeman.
Grobstein, C.
    1988. Science and the Unborn. New York: Basic Books.
Guan, K., K. Nayerma, L. S. Maier, et al.
    2006. Pluripotency of spermatogonial stem cells from adult mouse testis.
        Nature 440 (27): 1199–1203.
Guinin, L. M.
    2001. Morals and primordials. Science 292:1659–60.
    2003. The set of embryo subjects. Nature Biotechnology 21:482–83.
Gurmankin, A. D., D. Sisti, and A. I. Caplan.
    2004. Embryo disposal practices in IVF clinics in the United States. Politics
        and the Life Sciences 22 (2): 4–8.
Hampton, T.
    2006. US stem cell research lagging. Journal of the American Medical Asso-
        ciation 295 (19): 2233–34.
Hoffman, D. I., G. L. Zellman, C. C. Fair, J. F. Mayer, J. G. Zeitz, W. E. Gibbons,
    and T. G. Turner Jr.
    2003. Cryopreserved embryos in the United States and their availability for
        research. Fertility and Sterility 79 (5): 1063–69.

Holden, C.

2006. Versatile sperm cells may offer alternative to embryos. Science 311 (March 31): 1850.

2007a. Stem cell candidates proliferate. Science 315 (Feb. 9): 761.

2007b. Stem cells: Controversial marrow cells coming into their own? Science 315 (Feb. 9): 760–61.

2007c. Stem cells: Data on adult stem cells questioned. Science 315 (March 2): 1207.

Holden, C., and G. Vogel.

2004. A technical fix for an ethical bind? Science 306 (Dec. 24): 2174–76. www.sciencemag.org.

Human eggs supply "ethical" stem cells.

2006. News. Nature 441 (June 29): 1038.

Human Embryonic Stem Cell Research Advisory Committee of the Board on Life Sciences of the Division on Earth and Life Studies and of the Board on Health Sciences Policy of the Institute of Medicine.

2007. Pre-publication Copy: 2007 Amendments to the National Academies' Guidelines for Human Embryonic Stem Cell Research. www.nap.edu/catalog/11871.html. Accessed March 14, 2007.

Human Fertilization and Embryology Authority.

2003. HFEA Code of Practice (6th Edition). www.hfea.gov.uk/docs/Code_of_Practice_Sixth_Edition-final.pdf.

Hwang, W. S., S. I. Roh, B. C. Lee, et al.

2005. Patient-specific embryonic stem cells derived from human SCNT blastocysts. Science 308:1777–83.

Hwang, W. S., Y. J. Ryu, J. H. Park, et al.

2004. Evidence of a pluripotent embryonic stem cell line derived from a cloned blastocyst. Science 303:1669–74.

Hyun, I., and K. W. Jung.

2006. Human research cloning, embryos, and embryo-like artifacts. Hastings Center Report 36 (5): 34–41.

Infertility Network.

2007. Stem cell research: UK-Newcastle to recruit egg donors. E-mail newsletter, Jan. 17, 2007. Available on request from Info@infertilitynetwork.org and Infertilitynetwork@yahoogroups.com.

International Society for Stem Cell Research.

2006. Guidelines for the conduct of human embryonic stem cell research. Draft, June 30. www.isscr.org/StaticContent/StaticPages/ISSCRTaskForceGuidelinesDRAFT6-30-06.pdf.

Jarmulowicz, M.

1990. Letters: Ethics, science, and embryos. Tablet 3 (Feb. 10): 181.

Kahn, J.

2004. Can health policy improve our understanding of the moral status of the human embryo? Presentation at the conference "Is It Possible to Say When

Human Life Begins? Can Ethical, Legal, and Biological Conceptions of the Human Embryo Converge?" July 14, La Jolla, CA, sponsored by the Center for Ethics in Science and Technology, the Burnham Institute, and the San Diego Science and Technology Council.

Kahn, J. P.
2006. What happens when politics discovers bioethics? Hastings Center Report 36 (3): 10.

Kass, L.
2002. President's Council on Bioethics: Chairman's vision. Jan. 17. bioethic-sprint.bioethics.gov/about/chairman.html or www.bioethics.gov. Accessed Jan. 10, 2007.

King, R. G.
1992. Los Angeles six months after. Los Angeles Times, Nov. 23, Metro, B6.

Klock, S. C.
2004. Embryo disposition: The forgotten "child" of in vitro fertilization. International Journal of Fertility 49 (1): 19–23.

Knowles, L. P.
2000. International perspectives on human embryo and fetal tissue research. In: National Bioethics Advisory Commission, ed. Ethical Issues in Human Stem Cell Research, vol. 2, Commissioned Papers, H1–22. Washington, DC: National Bioethics Advisory Commission.

Landry, D. W., and H. A. Zucker.
2004. Embryonic death and the creation of human embryonic stem cells. Journal of Clinical Investigation 114 (9): 1184–86.

Lanza, R. P., H. Y. Chung, J. J. Yoo, et al.
2002. Generation of histocompatible tissues using nuclear transplantation. Nature Biotechnology 20 (July): 689–96. http://biotech.nature.com.

Lebacqz, K.
2001. On the elusive nature of respect. In: S. Holland, K. Lebacqz, and L. Zoloth, eds. The Human Embryonic Stem Cell Debate: Science, Ethics, and Public Policy. Cambridge, MA: MIT Press.

Liao, S. M.
2005. Rescuing human embryonic stem cell research: The blastocyst transfer method. American Journal of Bioethics 5 (6): 8–16.

Loring, J. F., and C. Campbell.
2006. Intellectual property and human embryonic stem cell research. Science 311:1716–17.

Marquis, D.
2006. Abortion and the beginning and end of human life. Journal of Law, Medicine and Ethics 34 (1): 16–25.

Martin, G. R.
1981. Isolation of a pluripotent cell line from early mouse embryos cultured in medium conditioned by teratocarcinoma stemcells. Proceedings of the National Academy of Science U.S.A. 78 (12): 7634–38.

McCormick, R. A.
   1991. Who or what is the pre-embryo? Kennedy Institute of Ethics Journal
   1 (1): 1–15.
McHugh, P. R.
   2004. Zygote and "clonote": The ethical use of embryonic stem cells. New
   England Journal of Medicine 351 (3): 209–11.
Melton, D. A., G. Q. Daley, and C. G. Jenning.
   2004. Altered nuclear transfer in stem-cell research: A flawed proposal. New
   England Journal of Medicine 351 (27): 2791–92.
Meyer, J. R.
   2000. Human embryonic stem cells and respect for life. Journal of Medical
   Ethics 26:166–70.
Millan, M. T., J. A. Shizuru, P. Hoffman, et al.
   2002. Mixed chimerism and immunosuppressive drug withdrawal after HLA-
   mismatched kidney and hematopoietic progenitor transplantation. Transplantation 73 (9): 1386–91.
Moreno, J., and S. Berger.
   2006. Taking stem cells seriously. American Journal of Bioethics 6 (5): 6–7.
Murray, F., and D. Spar.
   2006. Bit player or powerhouse? China and stem-cell research. New England
   Journal of Medicine 355 (12): 1191–94.
National Academies.
   2007a. Human Embryonic Stem Cell Research Advisory Committee.
   http://dels.nas.edu/bls/stemcells/guidelines.shtml. Accessed Jan. 11, 2007.
   2007b. Understanding Stem Cells: An Overview of the Science and Issues
   from the National Academies. Washington, DC: National Academies
   Press. www.nationalacademies.org/stemcells. Accessed March 18, 2007.
National Bioethics Advisory Commission.
   1999. Ethical Issues in Human Stem Cell Research. Vol. 1. Report and Recommendations of the National Bioethics Advisory Commission. Rockville,
   MD: National Bioethics Advisory Commission.
   2000. Ethical Issues in Human Stem Cell Research. Vol. 2. Commissioned
   Papers. Rockville, MD: National Bioethics Advisory Commission.
National Research Council/Institute of Medicine. Committee on the Biological
   and Biomedical Applications of Stem Cell Research.
   2002. Stem Cells and the Future of Regenerative Medicine. Washington, DC:
   National Academies Press.
Nelson, L. J., and M. J. Meyer.
   2005. Confronting deep moral disagreement: The President's Council on
   Bioethics, moral status, and human embryos. American Journal of
   Bioethics 5 (6): 33–42.
Normile, D.
   2006. Stem cell research: South Korea picks up the pieces. Science
   312:1298–99.

Owen-Smith, J., and J. McCormick.
    2006. An international gap in human ES cell research. Nature Biotechnology
        24 (4): 391–92.
Pearson, H.
    2006. Early embryos can yield stem cells . . . and survive. Nature 442 (24): 858.
Peterson, J. C.
    2003. Is a human embryo a human being? In: B. Waters and R. Turner, eds.
        God and the Embryo: Religious Voices on Stem Cells and Cloning. Wash-
        ington, DC: Georgetown University Press.
Philpott, S.
    2005. Eggs, lies and compromise. American Journal of Bioethics 5 (6): 1–3.
Pontifical Academy for Life.
    2000. Declaration "On the Production and the Scientific and Therapeutic Use
        of Human Embryonic Stem Cells." Aug. 25. www.petersnet.net/browse/
        3021.htm. Accessed Jan. 10, 2007.
President's Council on Bioethics.
    2003. Staff working paper for October 17, 2003, meeting. www.bioethics
        .gov/transcripts/oct03/index.html.
    2004a. Dec. 2–3, 2004 meeting agenda. www.bioethics.gov/transcripts/
        dec04/session6.html. Accessed March 17, 2007.
    2004b. Monitoring Stem Cell Research. Prepublication version. Jan.
        www.bioethics.gov/reports/stemcell/index.html. Accessed Jan. 10, 2007.
    2005. White Paper: Alternative Sources of Human Pluripotent Stem Cells.
        May. http://bioethicsprint.bioethics.gov/reports/white_paper. Accessed
        Jan. 10, 2007.
Reeve, C.
    2004. Christopher Reeve keynote address transcript. Oct. 10. Presented at the
        50th anniversary of the Rehabilitation Institute of Chicago. www.ric.org/
        about/reeve_transcript.php. Accessed Jan. 10, 2007.
Reichardt, T., D. Cyranoski, and Q. Schiermeier.
    2004. Religion and science: Studies of faith. Nature 432:666–69.
Romney, L.
    2006. State takes lead in stem cell efforts. Los Angeles Times, July 21,
        B1, 7.
Saletan, W.
    2004. Monster farming: The creepy solution to the stem cell debate. Slate,
        Dec. 5. http://slate.msn.com/id/211–0670.
Sandel, M. J.
    2004. Embryo ethics: The moral logic of stem cell research. New England
        Journal of Medicine 351 (3): 207–9.
Savulescu, J., and R. Saunders.
    2006. The "Hinxton Group" considers transnational stem cell research. Hast-
        ings Center Report 36 (3): 49. To be available at www.hopkinsmedicine
        .org/bioethics.

Scadden, D. T.
2006. The stem-cell niche as an entity of action. Nature 441:1075–79.

Schwartz, P. H., and S. B. Rae.
2006. An approach to the ethical donation of human embryos for harvest of stem cells. Reproductive BioMedicine Online 12 (6): 771–75. www.rbmonline.com/Article/2332.

Schwartz, R. S.
2006. The politics and promise of stem cell research. New England Journal of Medicine 355 (12): 1189–91.

Scott, C. T.
2006. Stem Cell Now: From the Experiment that Shook the World to the New Politics of Life. New York: Pi Press.

Shamblott, M. J., J. Axelman, S. Wang, E. M. Bugg, J. W. Littlefield, P. J. Donovan, P. D. Blumenthal, G. R. Higgins, and J. D. Gearhart.
1998. Derivation of pluripotent stem cells from cultured human primordial germ cells. Proceedings of the National Academies of Sciences 95: 13726–31.

Siegel, A. W.
2000. Locating convergence: Ethics, public policy, and human stem cell research. In: National Bioethics Advisory Commission, ed. Ethical Issues in Human Stem Cell Research, vol. 2, Commissioned Papers, J1–11.

Snyder, E. Y., and J. F. Loring.
2006. Beyond fraud: Stem-cell research continues. New England Journal of Medicine 354 (4): 321–24.

Steinbock, B.
2006. The morality of killing human embryos. Journal of Law, Medicine and Ethics 34 (1): 26–34.

Stolberg, S. G.
2006. First Bush veto maintains limits on stem cell use. New York Times, July 20.

Strelchenko, N., O. Verlinsky, V. Kukharenko, and Y. Verlinsky.
2004. Morula-derived human embryonic stem cells. Reproductive BioMedicine Online 9 (6): 623–29.

Strober, S., R. J. Lowsky, J. A. Shizuru, J. D. Scandling, and M. T. Millan.
2004. Approaches to transplantation tolerance in humans. Transplantation 77 (6): 932–36.

Strong, C.
2005. Obtaining stem cells: Moving from Scylla toward Charybdis. American Journal of Bioethics 5 (6): 21–23.

Thomson, J. A., J. Itskovitz-Elder, S. S. Shapiro, M. A. Waknitz, J. J. Swiergiel, V. S. Marshall, and J. M. Jones.
1998. Embryonic stem cell lines derived from human blastocysts. Science 282:1145–47.

Vogel, G.
   2006a. Four genes confer embryonic potential. Science 313:27.
   2006b. International standards proposed for stem cell work. Science 313:26.

Vogelstein, B., B. Alberts, and K. Shine.
   2002. Please don't call it cloning! Science 295 (Feb. 15): 1237.

Wade, N.
   2006. Science Academy creating panel to monitor stem-cell research. New
       York Times, Feb. 16, A21.

Wang, H., S. C. Hung, S. T. Peng, C. C. Huang, H. M. Wei, Y. J. Guo, Y. S. Fu,
   M. C. Lai, and C. C. Chen.
   2004. Mesenchymal stem cells in the Wharton's jelly of the human umbilical
       cord. Stem Cells 22:1330–37.

Warnock, M.
   1985/1992. A Question of Life: The Warnock Report on Human Fertilization
       and Embryology. Oxford: Blackwell.

Weiss, M. G., and A. L. Basham.
   1995. Hinduism. In: W. T. Reich, ed. Encyclopedia of Bioethics. rev. ed. New
       York: Simon and Schuster.

Weissman, I. Stem cell research: Paths to cancer therapies and regenerative medicine. Journal of the American Medical Association 294 (11): 1359–66.

Wilmut, I., A. E. Schnieke, J. McWhir, A. J. Kind, and K. H. S. Campbell.
   1997. Viable offspring derived from fetal and adult mammalian cells. Nature
       385 (6619): 810–13.

Young, E. W. D.
   2001. Ethical issues: A secular perspective in the human embryonic stem cell
       debate. In: S. Holland, K. Lebacqz, and L. Zoloth, eds. Science, Ethics, and
       Public Policy. Cambridge, MA: MIT Press.

Epilogue

Kristen Renwick Monroe and Ted Wrigley

It is difficult to write a "last word" on an area in which scientific and political events are occurring so rapidly, particularly one such as embryonic
stem cell research, which raises difficult ethical issues that may extend
beyond the normal philosophical purview of medicine, law, and religion.
Experts and lay people alike are understandably confused and unsure
about policy that touches on some of their most deeply help ethical and
religious concerns, yet holds tremendous potential for scientific breakthroughs and medical improvements in the quality of life for countless
individuals, as laid out by Bryant and Schwartz in chapter 1.[1] The stakes
are high, in ethical terms as well as in medical and economic terms. Given
the breadth and complexity of the issues, there are questions we have not
been able to address fully in this volume. For instance, we have touched
only partially on the tremendous economic potential of stem cell research, which is creating an incentive toward speculation on the part
of individuals, companies, various U.S. states, and even entire nations.
Chapter 7, by Golub, looked at the attempts by California and several
other states to create funding opportunities in lieu of federal support, but
U.S. states are not the only places gambling that a huge investment of
cash will yield huge proceeds. South Korea, Britain, and China each have
strong research programs with none of the restrictions imposed in the
United States by the federal government. Further, as Goldstein and
Miller both suggest briefly in chapters 5 and 8, researchers will go where
they can find the funding and resources they need to do their work, and

this will in turn draw talent away from other related fields. Restrictions on stem cell research in the United States thus are likely to set back biomedical progress in this nation across the board and to feed back into the way the scientific research is done. Perhaps because of this, stem cell research is already on track to become a matter of national pride and identity. The competition between the United States and Soviet Union over space flight in the 1960s had an incalculable fallout in the public imagination; stem cell research, where scientists are perceived to be delving into the nature of life itself, can hardly do less. There is fodder here to feed public political debate for decades.

Perhaps the most difficult factor to address is the political and ethical significance of the development of new techniques and technologies, some of which carry the potential to transform, or even obviate, many ethical questions that we ask today. A dramatic illustration of this comes from recent research (Chung et al. 2006) indicating that it might be possible to extract new stem cell lines without risk to any potential life. In this procedure—a procedure that, to the best of our knowledge, has not been replicated and has been attempted only with mice—a single cell is carefully removed from the eight cells of a blastomere. The remaining cells can go on to produce a normal, healthy fetus. The extracted cell, on the other hand, has no potential for developing into a viable embryo, and so no harm comes from using it to generate stem cells.[2] If future scientific work replicates these findings in humans, then perhaps religious concerns over the destruction or continuous harvesting of a viable embryo would no longer apply. It is impossible to intuit which of the current ethical issues these new procedures will resolve and what future ethical questions these procedures themselves will in turn produce. It seems safe to predict, however, that political battles will continue to influence the public debate over stem cells, just as public discussions over earlier scientific discoveries influenced public debate on issues as diverse as smallpox inoculations, the polio vaccine, and fluoridated water.

So what is our intention in this volume? Although the senior editor is a political scientist, we have chosen not to focus on a political science analysis of how this important policy issue is playing out in political terms. Instead, we have tried to present the central issues in the public discussion over stem cells in a manner that is comprehensive but accessible to the general reader. The immediacy of the decisions confronting citizens and policy makers is simply too great not to provide such a service. In this volume, therefore, we have chosen to restrict ourselves to considering the relationship between religious, ethical, and scientific beliefs about stem cells and human life, because that is where the current political confrontations over restrictions and funding lie.

Our initial analysis suggests that the public debate—at least so far—is being miscast and shaped into terms that are unnecessarily confrontational. In an effort to clarify and move discussion from this confrontational mode, we began with a discussion of the technical, scientific issues involved in stem cell research (chapters 1 and 2, by Peter Bryant and Phil Schwartz). Next, we attempted to deconstruct the debate over the moral status of the blastocyst. Chapter 3, by Philip Nickel, did so by discussing in detail the moral standing of the blastocyst; chapter 8, by Ronald Miller, focused on an examination of the concept of personhood and our understanding of our responsibilities to others in a society. Nickel analyzed the various moral standards that can be applied to the stem cell question, ultimately suggesting that the most applicable standards are those applied to donated organs: showing a general respect for the wishes of the deceased and relatives without according any special rights and privileges to the organs now deprived of independent life. Miller, in his turn, placed personhood on an incremental scale, showing that the biological organism is developmental and that few of the attributes that we credit to an adult person apply. Jafari et al., in chapter 4, addressed this same issue from a religious rather than a biological perspective. These contributors examined different religious beliefs from around the world and showed that the particular concerns raised in this debate are not universally shared or generally accepted as true but rather belong to a handful of sects of the Christian faith. This fact remains largely ignored in public discussions of embryonic stem cell research, at least in the United States, but could have tremendous importance for the worldwide research on stem cells.

Lee Zwanziger (chapter 6) and Larry Goldstein (chapter 5) each looked at the relationship of government to science and technology. Zwanziger demonstrated that science is a good in and of itself, something to be promoted as a matter of policy, since it speaks to the health and welfare of the society at large. Goldstein pointed out that government funding is vital for basic research, which (unlike product development) reaps little reward for private investors and encourages a degree of transparency and collegiality in the process that would go against the interests of for-profit companies.

In general, these authors seem to suggest that the functional pragmatism of scientific investigation—which is often cast as moral relativism by its opponents—is faced off against a fundamentalist belief in the sanctity of life—seen by its opponents as mindless fanaticism. Several, in fact, doubt that this polarity can be easily overcome. Perhaps then, the concluding question we should raise—because it is fundamental to the problems being faced here—is one raised initially by Paul Silverman when he proposed this volume: If public discussion of stem cell research involves us in questions about the origins and nature of life, whose life are we asking about? Medicine as a discipline has always focused on the lives of those we see passing us on the street each day: our friends, family, and selves, among the multitude of others. This may lead medicine to a certain callousness toward those not included in the visible spectrum of humanity. As is well known, laboratory rats, guinea pigs, and rhesus monkeys have suffered the consequences of human medical advances since the beginning of medicine as a science. To the medical eye and imagination, a blastocyst sitting in a frozen storage container in a fertility clinic harbors a potential cure for a broad range of human misery among the living, and it would be a waste to dispose of it. To the religious fundamentalist eye, however, that same blastocyst is a life in its own right, one that should not be subjected to experimentation or manipulation. An important part of the public debate is focused on the potential for conscious life that the blastocyst represents.

The irony in this disagreement is that the fundamentalists have chosen a purely genetic description of humanity, while medicine has held to a more conventional description. A blastocyst has nothing in common with an adult human except for the strands of DNA that place it in the human species and (in the assumption of some) a soul. The genetic code is the only observable element that differentiates a human blastocyst from rats, rhesus monkeys, and other experimental animals, animals whose lives are not a concern in the fundamentalist perspective. Most medical practitioners, by contrast, take as fully human that which appears to be fully human, without too much consideration of what that means. If it has a human form, can talk, or can at least interact socially and respond in an intelligible way, then it is treated as human. Neither depiction of humanity is fully satisfactory, nor are these depictions even necessarily exclusive, but in the political world they have been constructed as deeply polarized opposites. Future debate on this issue must clarify and resolve this division if there is to be any hope of a satisfactory resolution to this issue. This volume, we hope, is a useful step in that direction.

NOTES

1. This is reflected in popular as well as scholarly journals—note the recent collaboration between *Scientific American* and the *Financial Times,* which covered a broad range of medical, economic, and political factors.

2. Similar efforts are underway using the cells harvested from amniotic fluid, umbilical cords, and other nongenerative sources of pluripotent stem cells.

REFERENCE

Chung, Y., et al.
    2006. Letter. *Nature* 439:216–19.

Contributors

PETER J. BRYANT, PhD, is a Professor in the UCI Department of Developmental and Cell Biology and is the Director of the UCI Interdepartmental Graduate Training Program in Molecular Biology, Genetics and Biochemistry. His research program includes the use of genetic methods in the fruit fly *Drosophila* to identify the genes involved in the control of stem cell division and differentiation in the nervous system. The human genome contains highly conserved counterparts of these *Drosophila* genes, and Dr. Bryant is investigating how they function in controlling the division and differentiation of human neural precursor cells. The work is leading to a better understanding of how stem cell development is controlled and will help in the effort to make stem cell therapy safer and more effective.

FANNY ELAHI is a PhD student in the Nuffield Department of Clinical Medicine at Oxford University. She is interested in molecular mechanisms critical for language-related brain development. The work done for her thesis is on protein interactions of FOXP2, a key molecular player in brain development necessary for linguistic functions.

LAWRENCE S. B. GOLDSTEIN, PhD, is Professor of Cellular and Molecular Medicine at the University of California, San Diego (UCSD), School of Medicine and an Investigator with the Howard Hughes Medical Institute (HHMI). His grants include funding from the National Institutes of Health (NIH), the Johns Hopkins ALS Center, and the High Q Foundation. He received his BA degree in biology and genetics from UCSD, received his PhD degree in genetics from the University of Washington, Seattle, and did postdoctoral research at the University of Colorado at Boulder and the Massachusetts Institute of Technology. He was Assistant, Associate, and Full Professor at Harvard University in the Department of Cellular and Developmental Biology and moved to UCSD and HHMI in 1993. His awards include a Senior Scholar Award from the Ellison Medical Foundation, an

American Cancer Society Faculty Research Award, and the Loeb Chair in Natural Sciences at Harvard University. His research focuses on the molecular mechanisms of movement inside neurons and the role of transport failures in neurodegenerative diseases. His lab has recently discovered important links between these transport processes and diseases such as Alzheimer's disease and Huntington's disease. Goldstein has played an active role in national science policy, serving on many public science advisory committees and testifying before Congress about NIH funding and stem cell research. He served as co-chair of the scientific advisory committee to the campaign for the Proposition 71 stem cell research initiative, which authorizes $3 billion in tax-free state bonds to fund stem cell research in California over the next ten years. As a cofounder and consultant of the biotechnology company Cytokinetics, he had an active role in private industry.

SIDNEY H. GOLUB, PhD, is Professor Emeritus at the University of California, Irvine (UCI). His scientific career in cancer immunology began at the Karolinska Institute, Stockholm, and continued at the University of California, Los Angeles, where he rose to Professor, Vice-Provost for Medical Sciences, and Interim Dean of the School of Medicine. In 1994 he became the Executive Vice Chancellor at the University of California, Irvine, and in 1999 the Executive Director of the Federation of American Societies for Experimental Biology. In 2003 he returned to UCI, where he is active in teaching and as a member of the UCI Stem Cell Research Center Advisory Committee. He is the chair of the UCI Embryonic Stem Cell Research Oversight (ESCRO) Committee.

MAHTAB JAFARI, PharmD, is an Assistant Professor and the Associate Director of Programs in Pharmaceutical Sciences in the College of Health Sciences at the University of California, Irvine (UCI). She received her doctorate of pharmacy from the University of California, San Francisco (UCSF) in 1994. She has held academic positions at the School of Pharmacy at UCSF and at the College of Medicine at UCI. She is a two-time recipient, as a course director in 2000 and as a course faculty member in 2002, of the National Institute of Healthcare Spirituality and Medicine Curricular Award. Through these grants, she developed courses and programs to teach belief systems in patient care to medical and pharmacy students. She has served as Director of the Cholesterol Clinic and Co-director of Cardiovascular Risk Reduction Program at the UCI Medical Center. Her current research focus is the impact of pharmaceuticals and botanicals on longevity pathways.

RONALD B. MILLER, MD, FACP, is Clinical Professor of Medicine Emeritus at the University of California, Irvine (UCI), where he founded the Renal Division of the Department of Medicine in 1968. After thirty years in academic and clinical nephrology, he became so concerned with the ethical issues in medicine that he founded the Program in Medical Ethics at UCI in 1989 and spent the 1989–90 year as a Visiting Scholar in Clinical Medical Ethics at the University of Chicago. He is a member of the UCI Stem Cell Research Center Advisory Committee and has spoken on the ethical issues of stem cell research, therapy, and public policy at UCI, the Whittier Law School, the National Kidney Foundation, and the University of California, San Diego.

KRISTEN RENWICK MONROE, PhD, is Professor of Political Science and Philosophy at the University of California, Irvine (UCI) and Director of the UCI Interdisciplinary Center for the Scientific Study of Ethics and Morality. Author or editor of nine books, she is best known for two books: *The Heart of Altruism*, a Pulitzer Prize nominee and 1997 recipient of the Best Book Award by the American Political Science Association (APSA), Section on Political Psychology; and *The Hand of Compassion*, a National Book Award nominee and winner of the Robert Lane Award and Honorable Mention for the Giovanni Sartori Award by APSA. Her most recent book is *Perestroika! The Raucous Revolution in Political Science* (Yale University Press, 2005), on methodological pluralism in social and political science. She has served as Vice-President of APSA and is the President (2007–8) of the International Society of Political Psychology.

PHILIP J. NICKEL, PhD, is Assistant Professor in the University of California, Irvine (UCI) Department of Philosophy and also teaches in UCI's School of Biological Sciences. He received his PhD in December 2002 from the University of California, Los Angeles. His research interest is in conceptualizing moral agency and moral belief from a social and developmental point of view. He is the author of papers on trust; on illness and vulnerability; and on the question of voluntary control over one's own beliefs.

SABA OZYURT is a PhD student in the Department of Political Science at the University of California, Irvine. Her interests are in political psychology, religion, and comparative politics. She is working on her dissertation on the political integration of Muslim women into Western society and is coauthor of a recent paper on gender equality in academia.

PHILIP H. SCHWARTZ, PhD, is a stem cell biologist who received two bachelor of science degrees at Seattle University and a PhD in neuroscience at the University of California, Los Angeles. He is Director of the Children's Hospital of Orange County Research Institute's National Human Neural Stem Cell Resource and is an Assistant Research Biologist at the University of California, Irvine's Developmental Biology Center.

JEROME S. TOBIS, MD, is Research Professor and Chairman Emeritus of the Department of Physical Medicine and Rehabilitation at the University of California, Irvine (UCI). He also served as Director of the Program on Geriatric Medicine and Gerontology, as Director of the Center for Complementary Medicine, as Chairman of the Medical Ethics Committee of the UCI Medical Center, and as a member of the Executive Board of the UCI Interdisciplinary Center for the Scientific Study of Ethics and Morality. Tobis is a Distinguished Alumnus of the Chicago Medical School, and he received the Distinguished Clinician Award of the American Academy of Physical Medicine and Rehabilitation. It was he and Paul Silverman who recommended that UCI hold the conference on stem cells that was held in May 2004 and that generated many of the papers in this volume.

TED WRIGLEY is a PhD candidate in the Political Science Department at the University of California, Irvine. His thesis is on deliberative democracy. He is working with Kristen Monroe on a paper on gender equality in academia and has done work on political psychology and on the methodology and philosophy of science.

LEE L. ZWANZIGER, PhD, is a staff member of the Food and Drug Administration (FDA)'s Center for Drug Evaluation and Research, Safety Policy and Communication and also works part time as a Visiting Assistant Professor of Science and Technology Studies at Virginia Polytechnic Institute and State University. She served previously as a staff member for the President's Council on Bioethics providing background research, and prior to that as a Study Director at the National Academies' Institute of Medicine on projects ranging from data privacy in health services research to the anthrax vaccine. In her earlier FDA connection, she worked in the Center for Drug Evaluation and Research on executive operations and staffing advisory committees. She came to the FDA from Peace Corps service, teaching basic sciences and medical ethics in Malawi's National School of Health Sciences.

Index

Text:	10/13 Sabon
Display:	Sabon
Indexer:	Barbara Roos
Compositor:	Binghamgon Valley Composition, LLC
Printer and binder:	Maple-Valley Manufacturing Group